Clinical Rounds in Hepatology

Virendra Singh · Akash Roy
Editors

Clinical Rounds
in Hepatology

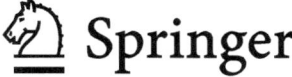 Springer

Editors
Virendra Singh
Department of Hepatology
Post Graduate Institute of Medical
Education and Research
Chandigarh, Punjab, India

Akash Roy
Department of Hepatology
Post Graduate Institute of Medical Education
and Research
Chandigarh, Punjab, India

ISBN 978-981-16-8447-0   ISBN 978-981-16-8448-7   (eBook)
https://doi.org/10.1007/978-981-16-8448-7

This Springer imprint is published by the registered company Springer Nature Singapore Pte Ltd.
The registered company address is: 152 Beach Road, #21-01/04 Gateway East, Singapore 189721,
Singapore

Contents

About the Editors and Contributors

About the Editors

Virendra Singh is working as Professor and Head of Hepatology at Postgraduate Institute of Medical Education and Research, Chandigarh, India, with more than 35 years of teaching experience. He completed his training in gastroenterology from the Institute of Medical Sciences, Banaras Hindu University, Varanasi, India, in 1988. He has published more than 135 papers in national as well as international journals. His areas of interest include ascites, post-paracentesis circulatory dysfunction, hepatorenal syndrome, hepatic regeneration in alcoholic hepatitis and cirrhosis, malignant hilar biliary obstruction, biliary injuries, and gastrointestinal tuberculosis.

Akash Roy is Senior Resident (Academic) at the Department of Hepatology, Post Graduate Institute of Medical Education and Research, Chandigarh. He did his MBBS from the Regional Institute of Medical Sciences, Imphal, and MD in internal medicine from NEIGRIHMS, Shillong. He has over 50 publications (national/international) to his credit and is the recipient of multiple awards in internal medicine and hepatology. His areas of interest include cirrhosis, alcoholic hepatitis, gut microbiota, and liver transplantation.

List of Contributors

Keisham Amarjit, MBBS, MD Department of Hepatology, Post Graduate Institute of Medical Education and Research, Chandigarh, Punjab, India

Harish Bhujade, MBBS, MD Department of Radiodiagnosis, Post Graduate Institute of Medical Education and Research, Chandigarh, Punjab, India

Ashim Das, MBBS, MD Department of Pathology, Post Graduate Institute of Medical Education and Research, Chandigarh, Punjab, India

Arka De, MBBS, MD, DM Department of Hepatology, Post Graduate Institute of Medical Education and Research, Chandigarh, Punjab, India

Prasanta Debnath, MBBS, MD, DM Department of Gastroenterology, TNMC and BYL Nair Charitable Hospital, Mumbai, India

Ajay Duseja, MBBS, MD, DM Department of Hepatology, Post Graduate Institute of Medical Education and Research, Chandigarh, Punjab, India

Akash Gandotra, MBBS, MD Department of Hepatology, Post Graduate Institute of Medical Education and Research, Chandigarh, Punjab, India

Naveen Kalra, MBBS, MD Department of Radiodiagnosis, Post Graduate Institute of Medical Education and Research, Chandigarh, Punjab, India

Yogendra Kumar, MBBS, MD Department of Hepatology, Post Graduate Institute of Medical Education and Research, Chandigarh, Punjab, India

Babu Lal Meena, MBBS, MD Department of Hepatology, Post Graduate Institute of Medical Education and Research, Chandigarh, Punjab, India

Rohit Mehtani, MBBS, MD Department of Hepatology, Post Graduate Institute of Medical Education and Research, Chandigarh, Punjab, India

Saurabh Mishra, MBBS, MD Department of Hepatology, Post Graduate Institute of Medical Education and Research, Chandigarh, Punjab, India

Madhumita Premkumar, MBBS, MD, DM Department of Hepatology, Post Graduate Institute of Medical Education and Research, Chandigarh, Punjab, India

Sahaj Rathi, MBBS, MD, DM Department of Hepatology, Post Graduate Institute of Medical Education and Research, Chandigarh, Punjab, India

Akash Roy, MBBS, MD Department of Hepatology, Post Graduate Institute of Medical Education and Research, Chandigarh, Punjab, India

Amandeep Singh, MBBS, MD Department of Hepatology, Post Graduate Institute of Medical Education and Research, Chandigarh, Punjab, India

Surender Singh, MBBS, MD Department of Hepatology, Post Graduate Institute of Medical Education and Research, Chandigarh, Punjab, India

Virendra Singh, MBBS, MD, DM Department of Hepatology, Post Graduate Institute of Medical Education and Research, Chandigarh, Punjab, India

Sunil Taneja, MBBS, MD, DM Department of Hepatology, Post Graduate Institute of Medical Education and Research, Chandigarh, Punjab, India

Arun Valsan, MBBS, MD Department of Hepatology, Post Graduate Institute of Medical Education and Research, Chandigarh, Punjab, India

U. V. U. Vamsidhar Reddy, MBBS, MD Department of Hepatology, Post Graduate Institute of Medical Education and Research, Chandigarh, Punjab, India

Aswath Venkitaraman, MBBS, MD Department of Hepatology, Post Graduate Institute of Medical Education and Research, Chandigarh, Punjab, India

Nipun Verma, MBBS, MD, DM Department of Hepatology, Post Graduate Institute of Medical Education and Research, Chandigarh, Punjab, India

Part I

Clinical Hepatology

Approach to Abnormal Liver Function Tests

Akash Gandotra, Akash Roy, and Virendra Singh

Case Vignette

A 46-year-old married male visits the outpatient department for elevated liver enzymes detected during annual check-up. He is an information technology professional with a sedentary lifestyle. He consumes alcohol (60–120 gm) on weekends without any history of binge. He has a history of hypertension and is on 40 mg of telmisartan. Family history was notable for coronary artery disease in his father. On examination, his height is 167 cm and body weight of 88 kg with a body mass index (BMI) of 32.83 g/m^2 and a waist circumference of 89 cm. He has a BP of 136/94 mmHg and pulse rate of 88/min. Per abdomen examination is remarkable for mild hepatomegaly.

Laboratory investigations revealed the following:

Parameter	Values	Parameter	Values
Haemoglobin	13.2	INR	1.1
Platelet count	150	HBsAg	NR
Total leukocyte count	7000	Anti-HCV	Negative
Total bilirubin (Direct)	1.2(0.8)	TG/LDL/HDL	282/94/12
AST	92	TSH	3.45
ALT	98	Urea	32
ALP	100	Creatinine	1.1
Albumin	3.5	HbA$_1$C	6.8

Abdominal ultrasound: Liver of 12.2 cm with regular margins and smooth surface and increased echogenicity. The spleen size was 8 cm, and the portal vein diameter was 9 mm. No presence of any free fluid.

A. Gandotra · A. Roy · V. Singh (✉)
Department of Hepatology, Post Graduate Institute of Medical Education and Research, Chandigarh, Punjab, India

© The Author(s), under exclusive license to Springer Nature Singapore Pte Ltd. 2022
V. Singh, A. Roy (eds.), *Clinical Rounds in Hepatology*,
https://doi.org/10.1007/978-981-16-8448-7_1

Transient Elastography (Fibroscan) showed liver stiffness measurement (LSM) 8.2 kpa with controlled attenuation parameter (CAP) 328.

Q. How would you describe the pattern of liver function tests in the given patient?

In the given patient, the liver function predominantly shows elevated liver transaminases which are typical for a hepatocellular pattern of cell injury. Hepatocellular injury is a disproportionate elevation of AST and ALT levels as compared to ALP. In cholestatic pattern of injury, there is a disproportionate increase in ALP level that is disproportionately elevated compared to the AST and ALT. Although traditionally described for drug-induced liver injury, the R-ratio (value) has been used to delineate the pattern of injury.

$$R \text{ value} = ALT/ULN \div AP/ULN$$

– Hepatocellular injury ($R \geq 5$ and ALT $>2\times$ ULN)
– Cholestatic injury ($R \leq 2$ and AP $>2\times$ ULN)
– Mixed injury ($5 > R > 2$ and ALT, AP both $>2\times$ ULN)

Q. What are the normal ranges for ALT?

Classically, the normal ranges for AST and ALT were defined as 8–40 and 5–35, respectively (Wróblewski F. The American journal of medicine. 1959). However, the recent guidelines suggest the normal ALT levels in healthy adults range from 29 to 33 IU/l for males and 19–25 IU/l for females, and levels beyond this should be evaluated (Kwo PY et al. ACG clinical guideline 2017).

Q. What are the historical pointers that need to be elicited while evaluating cases with elevated liver enzymes?

In a patient with suspicion of liver disease and persistently elevated aminotransferase levels a detailed history taking is the mandated first step: patient's history in detail.

• H/O anorexia, generalized weakness, low-grade fever indicated hepatocellular necrosis and are classically seen in viral hepatitis.
• H/O polyarthritis, arthralgia, rashes, and associated autoimmune conditions.
• H/O cholestasis (clay coloured stools, pruritis).
• History of alcohol use, intravenous drug usage, illicit substance usage, sexual promiscuity, tattooing, needle pricks, unsterilized shaving instrument sharing, and ear piercings.
• Detailed drug history with particular attention to complementary and alternative medicine intake.
• H/O chronic medical comorbidities (type 2 diabetes, hypertension, obesity, hyperuricemia, dyslipidaemia)
• H/O extrahepatic abnormalities include thyroid disorders, cardiac disorders, hypogonadism, and inflammatory bowel disease.

- Family history of chronic hepatitis, history of liver failure in siblings, liver disease in the family, and/or known death due to liver disease in the family and history of indirect hyperbilirubinemia if present.
- Family history of hepatic or non-hepatic cancers.

Q. What are the general examination assessments in the evaluation of a patient with elevated transaminases?
- Anthropometry (height, weight, BMI assessment, and recording of maximum premorbid body weight), thyroid examination, peripheral markers of dyslipidaemia
- Tattoo marks, evidence for intravenous drug usage, nail changes, and Kayser Fleischer rings
- Stigmata of chronic liver disease (palmar erythema, gynaecomastia, Duputeryan's contracture, parotid enlargement, paper money skin, testicular atrophy etc.)
- Signs for liver cell failure (icterus, ascites, hepatic encephalopathy)

Bonus Points
Bilirubin:
- **Normal range** for total bilirubin is usually up to 1.1 mg/dL of which nearly 70% is indirect/unconjugated.
- **Unconjugated hyperbilirubinaemia:** Indirect fraction ≥80% of total bilirubin seen classically in haemolytic disorders, hyperthyroidism, Gilbert's syndrome, Crigler-Najjar syndrome type I and II, Lucy-Driscoll syndrome.
- **Conjugated hyperbilirubinaemia:** Direct fraction ≥50% of total bilirubin and is usually seen in hepatocellular dysfunction or cholestasis.
- In cases of choledocholithiasis leading to bile flow obstruction, it is unusual for the bilirubin level to increase to more than 15 mg/dL because obstruction is usually incomplete and is <6.0 mg/dL.
- Conjugated bilirubin (water soluble) in extrahepatic cholestasis is excreted easily by the kidney. Thus, bilirubin excretion keeps pace with bilirubin production. Therefore, if bilirubin is higher than 25–30 mg/dL additional pathologies like associated haemolysis and renal failure should be looked for.

Q. Enumerate the causes of elevated transaminase levels

(a) **Hepatic causes of elevated transaminases:**

Pattern (AST>ALT): Alcoholic hepatitis, cirrhosis (of any aetiology), ischaemic hepatitis, congestive hepatopathy, acute Budd-Chiari syndrome, hepatic artery, and due to total parenteral nutrition (TPN).

Pattern ALT>AST: NASH, viral hepatitis (acute and chronic), drug-induced liver injury, toxin-induced hepatic damage, autoimmune hepatitis, metabolic liver disorders, sepsis-induced liver dysfunction.

(b) **Non-hepatic causes of elevated transaminases**

Rhabdomyolysis, cardiac injury, thyroid disease, macro-ASTemia, strenuous exercise, haemolysis, and adrenal insufficiency (Kwo PY et al. ACG clinical guideline 2017).

(Macro-ASTemia: A rare cause of isolated AST elevation is the presence of macro-AST in which there is a development of complexes of AST with immunoglobulins, which leads to its reduced clearance from the blood).

Q. What is the pattern of hepatic transaminase elevation in alcoholic hepatitis?

Since the alcohol-mediated damage leads to significant mitochondrial dysfunction, the rise in AST (present both in mitochondria and in cytosol) is higher than that of the ALT (confined to cytosol). Furthermore, alcoholics have pyridoxine deficiency. ALT is more sensitive to pyridoxine deficiency; hence ALT is comparatively lower. Consequently, in patients with alcoholic hepatitis, the AST: ALT ratio is usually greater than 1.5 and the AST increase is not more than 400 U/L.

Q. Describe in brief about alkaline phosphatase

Alkaline phosphatase (ALP) belongs to a group of hydrolytic enzymes which mediate the hydrolysis of phosphate esters. It is named alkaline as it acts at an alkaline pH.

Sources: Bone, placenta, intestine, and kidney as well as in liver Hence, if ALP is increased then the next step is to confirm its hepatic origin by assessing gamma-glutamyl transpeptidase levels. The hepatic alkaline phosphatase is synthesized by the bile duct epithelial cells and the synthesis increases when there is biliary obstruction. Therefore, a raised alkaline phosphatase can indicate obstruction of relatively few small bile ducts which are insufficient to cause a rise in the serum bilirubin.

Hepatic Causes of Raised ALP

Cholestasis (Intrahepatic or extrahepatic)

Infiltrative liver disorder: Granulomatous disorders (tuberculosis, sarcoidosis), lymphoma, amyloid, metastatic cancers, fungal infections

Hyperthyroidism

Liver abscesses

Ductopenia/Vanishing bile duct syndrome

Cardiac failure

Hemophagocytic lymphohistiocytosis

Intrahepatic cholestasis of pregnancy

Q. What are the causes for low ALP?

- Hypothyroidism
- Wilson's disease
- Haemolysis
- Congenital hypophosphatasia
- Aceruloplasminemia

Q. What are the causes for raised GGT (Gamma-glutamyl Transferase/ Transpeptidase)?

- Intrahepatic or extrahepatic biliary obstruction (highly elevated)
- Acute hepatitis (modest elevations)
- Heavy sustained alcohol consumption
- Drugs (enzyme inducers): Phenytoin and phenobarbitone
- Acute and chronic pancreatitis
- Prostatic adenocarcinoma (Vroon DH, Israili Z. 2011)

Further Reading

Kamath PS. Clinical approach to the patient with abnormal liver test results. Mayo Clin Proc. 1996;71(11):1089–95. Elsevier

Acute Liver Failure

Amandeep Singh, Akash Roy, and Virendra Singh

Case Vignette A 22-year-old male came with a history of fever which was low grade for 5 days associated with nausea and malaise. The family members noted yellowish discoloration of his eyes for last 3 days. The fever has subsided over the last 24 h but the patient has developed drowsiness and irrelevant behaviour for 1 day. There is no history of similar illnesses in the past. No history of alcohol intake, blood transfusions, major surgeries, tattooing, or illicit drug intake. No history of similar illnesses in the family or in a nearby locality. On clinical examination, he is deeply icteric. Per abdominal examination is unremarkable. There is presence of asterixis.

Laboratory investigations of blood revealed the following:

Parameter	Values	Parameter	Values
Hemoglobin	11	INR	2.1
Platelet count	150	HBsAg	NR
Total leukocyte count	14000	Anti-HCV	Neg
Total bilirubin (Direct)	7 (5.2)	Procalcitonin	1
AST	765	S Na/K	125/4.3
ALT	1230	Albumin	3.6
ALP	89	Urea/Creatinine	40/1.1
Ig M HAV: Negative			
ANA: Negative			
IgM HEV: Positive			

A. Singh · A. Roy · V. Singh (✉)
Department of Hepatology, Post Graduate Institute of Medical Education and Research, Chandigarh, Punjab, India

© The Author(s), under exclusive license to Springer Nature Singapore Pte Ltd. 2022
V. Singh, A. Roy (eds.), *Clinical Rounds in Hepatology*, https://doi.org/10.1007/978-981-16-8448-7_2

Q. Define Acute Liver Injury and Acute Liver Failure
- **Acute Liver Injury:** Liver dysfunction and coagulopathy (INR>1.5) but no alteration of consciousness.
- **Acute Liver Failure:** Jaundice with coagulopathy INR≥1.5 with any degree of hepatic encephalopathy in a patient with no pre-existing chronic liver disease.

Q. What are the exceptions to the diagnosis of Acute Liver Failure?
Traditionally, patients with background chronic disease are not included in the definition of ALF. However, acute presentations of certain diseases (**Acute Wilsons' Disease, Acute Autoimmune Hepatitis, Acute HBV, and Acute Budd Chiari Syndrome**) are considered as exceptions and included in the definition of ALF.

Q. Classify ALF on the basis of Jaundice to Encephalopathy interval
- Hyperacute: Up to 7 days
- Acute: 7–28 days
- Subacute: 28 days to 26 weeks

Q. What are the common causes of Acute Liver Failure?
Evidence based on Western literature suggests Acetaminophen overdose as the most common cause of ALF, whereas reports from developing nations report viral hepatitis (HAV, HEV) as the most common cause of ALF. Overall, the most common causes include:

- Acetaminophen overdose
- Drug-induced liver injury
- Hepatotropic viruses: HAV, HEV, and HBV
- Autoimmune hepatitis
- Budd Chiari syndrome
- Ischaemic hepatitis
- Pregnancy-specific liver disease (Acute fatty liver of pregnancy)

Q. What are the King's College Criteria for Acute Liver Failure?
The King's College criteria were originally devised in 1989 to determine indicators of poor prognosis in patients with ALF, which would prioritize the need for liver transplantation (Table 2.1).

Table 2.1 King's College Criteria for emergency liver transplantation

Paracetamol and hyperacute aetiologies	Non-paracetamol
Arterial pH <7.30 after resuscitation	INR >6.5
Lactate >3 mmol/L	Any three of the following:
Any three of the following:	Indeterminate aetiology
INR >6.5	Age <10 or >40
HE Grade 3	Jaundice to encephalopathy >7 days
Serum creatinine >300 μmol/l	Bilirubin >300 μmol/l
	INR >3.5

Q. What Are the ALFED Model and Clinical Prognostic Indicator System in Acute Liver Failure?

ALFED (ALF Early Dynamic Model) score: Most scores for prognostic assessment are static, the ALFED score provides a dynamic assessment system for the determination of outcomes in ALF (Table 2.2).

Based on the total score, patients stratified into three risk categories as follows (Table 2.3).

Clinical Prognostic Indicators (CPI): This score is predominantly used with viral hepatitis as the aetiology and is useful where viral hepatitis forms the predominant aetiology. The score consists of the following parameters:

- Age ≥ 50 years
- Jaundice encephalopathy interval >7 days
- Grade 3 or 4 encephalopathy at presentation
- Presence of cerebral oedema
- PT ≥ 35 seconds
- Creatinine ≥ 1.5 mg/dl

Presence of 3 of 6 CPI is considered optimum for differentiating between survivors and non-survivors according to this score.

(Dhiman RK et al. Early indicators of Prognosis in Fulminant Hepatic Failure: An assessment of the Model for End-Stage Liver Disease (MELD) and King's College Hospital Criteria. Liver Transpl. 13:814-821, 2007)

Table 2.2 ALFED model for prediction of outcomes in ALF

Variables over 3 days	Score assigned
HE, persistent or progressed to grade >2	2
INR, persistent or progressed to level ≥ 5	1
Arterial ammonia, persistent or increased to level ≥ 123 umol/l	2
Serum bilirubin, persistent or increased to level ≥ 15 mg/dl	1

(Kumar R et al. Prospective. Derivation and validation of Early dynamic model for predicting outcome in patients with acute liver failure. Gut 2012; 61:1068)

Table 2.3 Risk stratification based upon ALFED model

Score	Risk status	Expected mortality (%)
0–1	Low	2.6
2–3	Moderate	19
4–6	High	88

Q. What are the other scoring systems in the assessment of Acute Liver Failure?

Multiple other scoring systems have been used to ascertain prognosis in acute liver failure. These include:

Clichy criteria: Also known as the Beaujon-Paul Brousse criteria. Its primary usefulness lies in identifying patients for emergency liver transplantation (HE stage ≥3 or Factor V levels <20% or <30% depending upon age).

MELD score: Although classically used for listing for patients for Liver transplant and outcomes after TIPSS, in patients with ALF a MELD of >33 is associated with poor prognosis and imminent need for liver transplantation.

ALFSG Index (Acute liver failure study group index): This index was devised to predict transplant-free survival and is a continuous predictive model. It includes Grade of HE, aetiology of liver failure, bilirubin levels, INR, and vasopressor requirement.

Q. What is the prognostic role of ammonia measurement in Acute Liver Failure?

Levels of ammonia are raised in cases with ALF as the capacity of the hepatocytes to metabolize ammonia to urea is overwhelmed. High levels of ammonia have been postulated as a possible prognostic indicator in patients with ALF with individual variations of cut-off level reported in studies. Bhatia et al. suggested a cut off of 124 $u$mol/L for mortality prediction, whereas Li et al. identified a cut-off of 122.5 $u$mol/L.

(Sheikh MF et al. Hepatology. 2019 and Li et al. Turk J Gastroenterol. 2021).

Q. What are the management principles in cases with Acute Liver Failure?

General Management Measures and management of raised intracranial pressure:

- Minimal stimulation.
- Nurse in a quiet environment with elevation of the head end of bed.
- Frequent neurological evaluation (Pupillary reflexes, deep tendon reflexes).
- Optic nerve sheath diameter assessment (4 hourly).
- Mechanical ventilation if HE>2 (West Haven Criteria).
- Adequate sedation once mechanically ventilated: Choice of Sedative: Propofol
- Target serum sodium 145–155 mEq/L: Corrections to be adjusted with Hypertonic saline.
- Use of Lactulose.
- Sustained surges in ICP (>25 mmHg) or development of clinical signs should be treated by a bolus of hypertonic saline (200 ml, 2.7% or 20 ml, 30%) or intravenous mannitol (150 ml, 20%) given over 20 min.
- Hyperventilation to maintain a target PCO2 of 25–30 mm Hg.

Infections

Surveillance for infections periodically with chest X-ray and site surveillance cultures.

Prophylactic antibiotics can be used if there is evidence of:

- Grade III/IV HE
- SIRS

Antifungals to be considered in presence of prolonged stay and onset of multiple organ failures.

Hemodynamic stabilization

Fluid resuscitation using normal saline or 5% albumin.

Targets of fluid replacement:

- MAP: 60–65 mm of Hg
- Urine Output: 0.5 ml/kg/hour
- Arterial lactate: <2 mmol/L

Coagulopathy

FFP/Platelet transfusion only if:

- Platelet count <20000/μL
- Active bleeding
- Before invasive procedure

Q. What are the aetiology-specific measures in Acute Liver Failure?

Etiology-specific measures

1. NAC-Acetaminophen and non-Acetaminophen ALF
   *Dose and administration of NAC in ALF
   Loading dose: 150 mg/kg I.V. in 5% dextrose over 15 min
   Maintenance dose: 50 mg/kg I.V. given over 4 h followed by 100 mg/kg I.V. administered over 16 h or 6 mg/kg/hr for 5 days.
2. Hepatitis B: HBV-specific therapy (Tenofovir, entecavir)
3. Herpes simplex hepatitis: Acyclovir
4. Cytomegalovirus hepatitis: Ganciclovir/Valganciclovir
5. Autoimmune hepatitis: Corticosteroids (low grade of HE; Unlikely to benefit once HE>3)
6. Mushroom poisoning: Penicillin-G/Silibinin
7. Pregnancy related (AFLP/HELLP): Delivery of foetus

Q. What is Optic Nerve Sheath Diameter (ONSD) and what is it's use in ALF?

The optic nerve has a sheath that is continuous with the dura mater of the brain. The subarachnoid space of the optic nerve sheath communicates with the brain and the subarachnoid space. Therefore, the optic nerve sheath diameter (ONSD) can be influenced by changes in the pressure of cerebrospinal fluid in the cranial cavity. ONSD is measured by an ultrasound probe placed on the eyes. A linear correlation between ICP and ONSD measurements has been reported with a cut-off value of >5.2 mm for ICP greater than 20 mmHg.

Q. What is the role of Plasmapheresis in Acute Liver Failure?

Plasmapheresis has a potential role in the management of ALF both as a bridge to transplant as well as a modality when transplant is not an option. The initial landmark study of plasmapheresis on ALF showed an increase in transplant-free survival. Further studies have shown varied results with improvement in biochemical parameters as well as improvement in survival.

Plasmapheresis in ALF landmark paper: (Larsen et al. High-volume plasma exchange in patients with acute liver failure: An open randomised controlled trial. J Hepatol. 2016)

Key Points:
- Open labelled randomized control trial.
- Number of patients: $n = 182$ (Plasma exchange + SMT 92, SMT 90).
- **Plasma exchange volume (High volume plasmapharesis):** 15% of ideal body weight (representing 8–12 L per day per procedure); patient plasma was removed at a rate of 1–2 L per hour with replacement with fresh frozen plasma in equivalent volume.
- Duration: HVP procedure was undertaken on three consecutive days but with no fixed time interval between each treatment.
- Results:
- HVP increases transplant-free survival after 3 months, and maximal effect of HVP was achieved in patients who did not undergo emergency transplantation.
- Overall hospital survival was 58.7% for patients treated with high volume plasma exchange vs 47.8% for control group HR: 0.56 (95%CI: 0.36–0.86), $P<0.01$).

Further Reading

Wendon J, et al. EASL clinical practical guidelines on the management of acute (fulminant) liver failure. J Hepatol. 2017;66(5):1047–81.

O'Grady J. Timing and benefit of liver transplantation in acute liver failure. J Hepatol. 2014;60(3):663–70.

Clinical Approach to Hepatitis B

Sunil Taneja, Akash Roy, and Virendra Singh

Case Vignette A 33-year-old male presented to the outpatient setting with new-onset malaise, low-grade fever, and progressive yellowish discoloration of eyes and urine. He gives a family history of hepatitis B in one of his siblings. There is no significant history of intravenous drug usage, blood transfusion, unsafe needle practices, tattooing, ear piercings, or outbreaks in the locality. On general examination, he had deep icterus. Per abdominal examination was unremarkable.
  Laboratory investigations revealed the following:

Parameter	Values	Parameter	Values
Hemoglobin	8.2	INR	1.3
Platelet count	154	HBsAg	Reactive
Total leukocyte Count	7000	Anti-HCV	Negative
Total bilirubin (Direct)	12 (8)	HBV DNA	5×10^4 IU/ml
AST	126	HBeAg/Anti-HBe	Neg/Neg
ALT	165	Urea	32
ALP	122	Creatinine	1.1
Albumin	3.5	AFP	6.8
IgM HAV	Neg	IgM HEV	Neg

Abdominal ultrasound: Liver of 12 cm with regular margins and smooth surface. The spleen size was 9 cm, and the portal vein diameter was 9 mm. No presence of any free fluid.

S. Taneja · A. Roy · V. Singh (✉)
Department of Hepatology, Post Graduate Institute of Medical Education and Research, Chandigarh, Punjab, India

© The Author(s), under exclusive license to Springer Nature Singapore Pte Ltd. 2022
V. Singh, A. Roy (eds.), *Clinical Rounds in Hepatology*,
https://doi.org/10.1007/978-981-16-8448-7_3

Q. What are the classical stages of Chronic HBV infection and what are the current terminologies for the classification of disease states?

Any patient with HBsAg present for at least 6 months is designated as CHB. Classically HBV infection has been divided into 4 phases:

Phase	ALT	HBV DNA	HBeAg	Liver biopsy
Immune tolerant	Usually normal	Increased	Positive	Minimal inflammation
Immune active (Immune clearance)	Increased	Increased	Positive	Moderate inflammation
Immune control (Inactive CHB)	Normal	Low or undetectable	Negative	Minimal necroinflammation
Immune reactivation	Increased	Increased	Negative	Moderate to severe inflammation/fibrosis

These stages have been recently modified according to the EASL guidelines in 2017.

Phase	ALT	HBV DNA	HBeAg	Liver biopsy
HBeAg positive chronic infection	Usually normal	$>10^7$	Positive	Minimal inflammation
HBeAg positive chronic hepatitis	Increased	10^4–10^7	Positive	Moderate inflammation
HBeAg negative chronic infection	Normal	<2000	Negative	None
HBeAg negative chronic hepatitis	Increased	>2000	Negative	Moderate to severe inflammation/fibrosis

Q. What are the recommended cut-offs according to AASLD for upper limit of ALT?

The upper limits of normal (ULN) for ALT in healthy adults are reported to be 29–33 U/L for males and 19–25 U/L for females. However, for management of CHB, a ULN for ALT of 35 U/L for males and 25 U/L for females is preferably used.

Q. How is the prevalence of HBsAg-positive persons stratified?

The prevalence of HBsAg is highly variable according to regions:

- High prevalence: ≥8%
- Intermediate prevalence: 2–7%
- Low prevalence: <2%

Q. What are the recommended screening strategies for HBV?

According to the AASLD screening should be done in all persons born in countries with an HBsAg seroprevalence of ≥2%. Additionally, people with high risk for HBV as enumerated below should also be screened for HBsAg:

- Men involved in promiscuous relations with men.
- Intravenous drug users (IVDU).
- People living with HIV-AIDS.
- Household and sexual contacts of HBV infected persons.
- Persons requiring immunosuppressive therapy.
- Persons on hemodialysis.
- Blood donors.
- Chronic hepatitis C patients.
- Any patient with persistently elevated aminotransferase.
- Incarcerated persons.
- Pregnant women.
- Infants born to HBV infected mother.
- Travelers to countries with intermediate or high prevalence of HBV infection.
- Unvaccinated persons with diabetes who are aged 19–59 years (clinician discretion advised for unvaccinated adults with diabetes >60 years of age).

Q. A person is detected to have HBsAg negative, anti-HBs titer negative but has Anti-HBc total positive. What are the possible implications in such a scenario?
Anti-HBc total is a marker for prior exposure to HBV either. Most common scenario in which the given presentation can occur is previous exposure to HBV infection who has recovered from acute HBV infection earlier in life and anti-HBs titers have declined to undetectable levels. Few other clinical scenarios in which this pattern may be seen are in patients with chronically infected HBV for decades with recent HBsAg clearance, window phase of acute hepatitis B, and HBsAg mutations leading to false-negative HBsAg results.

Q. What is the principle of HBV therapy? Compare the AASLD and the EASL recommendations of treatment of Chronic Hepatitis B
In case an adult is chronically infected, there is an 8–20% risk of developing cirrhosis. Once cirrhosis sets in the 5-year risk of decompensated cirrhosis is 20% and risk of developing HCC is 2–5%. Hence, the primary goal of therapy for CHB is to reduce and prevent progression of liver disease. The ultimate endpoint of HBV therapy should be elimination of integrated DNA and cccDNA. However, this is difficult to achieve and hence surrogate markers are used of which HBsAg loss is most commonly used. However, in clinical practice this is rarely seen. Hence, easily monitorable parameters like HBV DNA suppression to undetectable levels and normalization of ALT are used to guide treatment. The decision to treat is complex and considers many variables including the phase of CHB, presence or absence of cirrhosis, and risk of disease progression. On account of these reasons, there are variations in the treatment strategies of various societies. The recommendations of the two primary societies are shown below:

Characteristics	AASLD (2018)	EASL (2017)
HBeAg positive	HBV DNA >20,000 IU/mL, ALT >2× ULN	HBV DNA >2000 IU/mL, ALT >ULN, and/or at least moderate liver, necroinflammation, or fibrosis
HBeAg negative	HBV DNA >2000 IU/mL, ALT >2× ULN	HBV DNA >2000 IU/mL, ALT >ULN, and/or at least moderate liver, necroinflammation, or fibrosis
Compensated cirrhosis	Adults with compensated cirrhosis even with low-level viremia (<2000 IU/mL) should be treated	Any detectable HBV DNA regardless of ALT levels
Decompensated cirrhosis	All patients	Any detectable HBV DNA regardless of ALT levels plus assessment of liver transplant *variation in text and recommendation
Additional patients who may require therapy	Adults >40, normal ALT, HBV, DNA ≥ 1,000,000 IU/mL with significant necroinflammation or fibrosis Family history of cirrhosis or HCC Extrahepatic manifestations	Patients with HBV DNA >20,000 IU/mL and ALT >2× ULN regardless of degree of fibrosis Family history of cirrhosis or HCC extrahepatic manifestations

Q. What are the recommendations for CHB in a patient who is pregnant?

All pregnancies in a CHB-positive mother should preferably have institutional delivery. Vaccination and hepatitis B immunoglobulin is recommended for the newborn. For mothers, those who have high levels of HBV DNA and who are HBeAg-positive are at an increased risk of transmission. Therefore, treatment in the third trimester is recommended in this group.

AASLD recommends therapy with TDF starting at 28 weeks with cut-offs for HBV DNA at >200,000 IU/mL.

EASL recommends therapy with TDF in patients with HBV DNA levels >200,000 IU/ml or HBsAg levels 4 log10 IU/ml starting at week 24–28 of gestation and continuing for up to 12 weeks after delivery. Additionally, EASL also recommends that patients who are pregnant and have evidence for fibrosis or cirrhosis should be treated with TDF.

Q. In cases with suspected Acute HBV infection, what are the recommendations of therapy?

Ninety-five percent of patients with acute HBV recover spontaneously. According to the EASL guidelines, only patients with severe acute hepatitis B (INR >1.5) or protracted course (marked jaundice >4 weeks) should be treated. The AASLD recommends antiviral treatment with Entecavir, TDF, or TAF for patients with acute hepatitis B who have acute liver failure or who have a protracted, severe course (Total bilirubin >3 mg/direct bilirubin >1.5 mg/dL), INR >1.5, encephalopathy, or ascites.

Q. How are HBV reactivation and flare defined?

In patients who are HBsAg positive HBV reactivation is defined by either of the following:

- ≥2 log increase in HBV DNA compared to the baseline level.
- HBV DNA ≥3 log (1000) IU/mL in a patient with a previously undetectable level.
- HBV DNA ≥4 log (10,000) IU/mL if the baseline level is not available.

In patients who are anti-HBc positive only HBV reactivation is defined as:

- HBV DNA is detectable
- Reverse HBsAg seroconversion occurs (reappearance of HBsAg)

A **hepatitis B flare** is defined as an ALT increase to ≥3 times the baseline level and >100 U/L.

Q. What are the differentiating points between Acute HBV and HBV Reactivation?

Characteristics	Reactivation of chronic HBV	Acute HBV
Clinical history	Known history or family history of CHB	Recently known exposure to HBV
Similarities	Prodrome ± Jaundice High transaminases	Prodrome ± Jaundice High transaminases
Ig M Anti-HBc	Low (<1:1000)	High (>1:1000)
HBV DNA	Highly increased (>10^5 copies/ml)	Increased (<10^5copies/ml)
Follow up	Have persistent HBsAg after 6 months	Loss of HBsAg in >95% on 6 months follow up
Histology	± Evidence of chronicity	No evidence of chronicity

Q. What are the recommended options for treatment of CHB?

Currently, there are two main treatment options for CHB patients, which include Nucleotide Analogues (NA) or Pegylated Interferon-alpha (Peg IFNa). The approved NA are classified as those having low barrier of resistance [lamivudine, adefovir dipivoxil, telbivudine] and those having a high barrier of resistance including entecavir (ETV), tenofovir disoproxil fumarate (TDF), and tenofovir alafenamide (TAF)].

The **preferred treatment options for patients for naive CHB according to EASL** are entecavir (ETV), tenofovir disoproxil fumarate (TDF), and tenofovir alafenamide (TAF).

Q. In which conditions are treatment with Entecavir/TAF Preferred over TDF?

Use of ETV or TAF over TDF is recommended only in certain specific situations which include:

Age >60 years
Bone disease

- Chronic steroid use or use of other medications that produce osteopenia
- History of fragility fracture
- Osteoporosis

Renal dysfunction

- eGFR <60 ml/min/1.73 m^2.
- Albuminuria [30 mg/24 h or moderate dipstick proteinuria].
- Low phosphate (<2.5 mg/dl).
- Hemodialysis.
  - TAF is preferred to ETV in patients with previous exposure to NAs.
  - ETV needs dose adjustment, dose needs to be adjusted if eGFR <50 ml/min.
  - TAF does not require dose adjustment in patients with age >12 years and body weight >35 kg with estimated creatinine clearance (CrCl) >15 ml/min or in patients with CrCl <15 ml/min who are receiving hemodialysis.

Q. What are the types of "Cure" in HBV infection?
Various types and definitions have been used to define cure in HBV treatment strategies which include:

Sterilizing cure: cccDNA not detected with no active transcription; Integrated DNA not detected.

Idealistic functional cure: cccDNA detected but no active transcription; Integrated DNA detection (±).

Realistic functional cure: cccDNA detected but no active transcription; Integrated DNA detected.

Attainable partial functional cure: cccDNA detected with low level of active transcription; Integrated DNA detected.

According to the recent EASL-AASLD endpoints in HBV guidance statements "functional HBV cure" is to be defined as durable hepatitis B surface antigen (HBsAg) loss (based on assays with a lower limit of detection ~0.05 IU/mL) with or without HBsAg seroconversion and undetectable serum HBV DNA after completing a course of treatment. Some key features at this stage include the presence of covalently closed circular (ccc) DNA is in liver in very small amounts or in a transcriptionally inactive state, with integrated HBV DNA being present (Cornberg M, et al J Hepatol. 2019).

Q. What are the potential surrogate markers for HBV cure?
HBsAg loss: Based upon currently available literature, the best surrogate of HBV functional cure is HBsAg loss confirmed on 2 occasions at least 6 months apart without the requirement for anti-HBs seroconversion plus undetectable HBV DNA and this should be considered as the primary treatment endpoint.

HBsAg levels: A declining HBsAg levels can be a predictor of potential HBsAg loss and is being evaluated as an exploratory marker. According to currently available literature, a reduced HBsAg level to a low level (<100 IU/mL of HBsAg) may reliably predict potential HBsAg loss on treatment.

It is important to note that HBsAg can be expressed both from cccDNA as well as integrated DNA with the latter being a more potent source in HBeAg-positive patients. This is important as newer biomarkers such as hepatitis B core-related antigen (HBcrAg) and HBV RNA may better reflect cccDNA status.

Further, this also has important therapeutic implications as patients on experimental agents targeting cccDNA may still be producing HBsAg from the integrated fragments even after cccDNA suppression.

Serum HBV RNA:

What is it? Serum HBV RNA is a mixture of intact, pregenomic (pg) and subgenomic, spliced RNA, and polyA-free RNA species.

What it corelates to?

- pgRNA, is the most direct measure of cccDNA transcriptional activity and according to recent literature, serum HBV pgRNA levels correlate with intrahepatic pgRNA and cccDNA content.
- It has been shown that detection of serum HBV RNA predicts posttreatment viral rebound after cessation of NA therapy.

What are the limitations? An important issue in the estimation of HBV RNA is avoiding cross detection of cross detect HBV DNA in addition to HBV RNA as well to characterize the type of HBV RNA that is measured (pgRNA/Total RNA/spliced RNA/truncated RNA).

HBcrAg

What is it? HBcrAg is a measure of the combined antigenic component reactivity from denatured HBeAg, HBV core antigen, and a truncated incompletely processed precore/core protein.

What does it measure?

- HBcrAg correlates well with intrahepatic cccDNA and its transcriptional activity.
- In cases with undetectable HBV DNA presence of HBcrAg indicates continued transcription from cccDNA.
- It has been shown to predict clinical relapse after stopping NA treatment and spontaneous or treatment-induced HBeAg seroconversion.
- HBcrAg levels are significantly higher in HBeAg-positive patients
- The primary potential utility of the use of HBcrAg are in newer treatment strategies that specifically target cccDNA.

What are the limitations? Although the sensitivity of current HBcrAg assays do seem adequate for monitoring untreated patients with high viremia, however, it needs to be improved for monitoring response on those patients who are already on antiviral treatment.

Additional markers:

- Quantitative hepatitis B core antibody (anti- HBc)
- Serum interferon-inducible protein-10 levels

Q. What are the novel therapeutic options in the treatment of HBV?
Besides established treatment strategies multiple novel mechanisms and treatment approaches are underway in the management of HBV. The various axis on which they act include:

- **Entry inhibitors:** NTCP inhibitor (Bulevertide)
- **Targeted endonuclease:** CRISPR/CAS9 system
- **HBx targeted therapy: Nitazoxanide**
- **TLR 7 agonist:** Vesatolimod
- **Checkpoint inhibitors:** Nivolumab
- **Core protein (Capsid) assembly modulators (CPAMs)**
- **cccDNA stabilizer**
- **HBsAg release inhibitors**
- **RNA interference and gene expression inhibitors**

Further Readings

Terrault NA, et al. Update on prevention, diagnosis, and treatment of chronic hepatitis B: AASLD 2018 hepatitis B guidance. Hepatology. 2018;67(4):1560–99.

Cornberg M, et al. Guidance for design and endpoints of clinical trials in chronic hepatitis B-Report from the 2019 EASL-AASLD HBV treatment endpoints conference. Hepatology. 2020;71(3):1070–92.

McMahon BJ. Epidemiology and natural history of hepatitis B. Semin Liver Dis. 2005;25(Suppl 1):3–8.

Practical Management of Chronic Hepatitis C

4

Akash Roy and Virendra Singh

Case Vignette

A 50-year-old female presented with gradually progressive, painless, generalized abdominal distension, and swelling of the legs for one-month duration. It was not associated with fever, periorbital puffiness, dyspnea, orthopnea, or reduced urine output. There was no history of jaundice, hematemesis, melena, or altered sleep pattern. The patient gives a history of reduced oral intake due to abdominal distension without any associated significant weight loss. There was no prior history of a similar illness. The patient was a teetotaler with no sexual promiscuity or high-risk behaviors. The patient also gave a history of blood transfusion around 30 years back during her first childbirth. She has a BMI of 24 kg/m². She was afebrile and had a BP 100/60 mm of Hg, pulse rate of 110/min, and respiratory rate of 16/min. Her physical exam revealed the presence of pallor and multiple spider angiomata. Per abdominal examination was remarkable for moderate grade ascites and a palpable spleen.

Laboratory investigations revealed the following:

Parameter	Values	Parameter	Values
Hemoglobin (g/dL)	8.2	INR	1.4
Platelet count (cu mm)	98	HBsAg	NR
Total leukocyte count	7000	Anti HCV	Positive
Total bilirubin (Direct)	1.8 (1.0)	Quantitative HCV RNA (IU/ml)/ Genotype	$8 \times 10^6/3$
AST (IU/dL)	98	S Na/K (mEq/dL)	132/4.3
ALT (IU/dL)	48	Urea (mg/dL)	32
ALP (IU/dL)	122	Creatinine (mg/dL)	1.1
Albumin (g/dL)	3.1	AFP (ng/mL)	6.8

A. Roy · V. Singh (✉)
Department of Hepatology, Post Graduate Institute of Medical Education and Research, Chandigarh, Punjab, India

© The Author(s), under exclusive license to Springer Nature Singapore Pte Ltd. 2022
V. Singh, A. Roy (eds.), *Clinical Rounds in Hepatology*, https://doi.org/10.1007/978-981-16-8448-7_4

Abdominal Ultrasound: Liver of 10 cm, nodular with irregular margin, spleen size of 13 cm, portal vein diameter of 14 mm, with moderate ascites

Q. What is the most probable diagnosis based upon the given clinical vignette?
Ans: HCV-related decompensated cirrhosis.

Q. What is the natural history of HCV infection?
Ans: Of those who develop acute HCV infection, 55–89% develop chronic HCV infection. Around 2–24% of patients with chronic hepatitis C develop cirrhosis over 20 years. Around 3% of patients with HCV cirrhosis will develop decompensating events each year. The risk of HCC in cirrhotics with HCV is 1–3% per year.

Q. What are the factors associated with the progression of hepatic fibrosis in Chronic HCV infection?
Ans:

Established risk factors	Possible associations	Not associated
Host factors	Male gender	Viral load
Older age of acquisition	Increased hepatic iron content	
Duration of infection		
Obesity		
Hepatic steatosis		
Severe necro-inflammation		
Insulin resistance		
White ethnicity		
Underlying Immune-suppression		
Viral factors		
HBV coinfection with Genotype 3		
HIV coinfection		
Environmental factors		
Alcohol consumption		
Marijuana use		
Smoking		

Q. Which population subgroups require screening for HCV Infection?
Ans:

High-risk exposure	High-risk behavior	Others
Hemodialysis	IV drug abuse	Persistently
Children born to HCV+ mother	High-risk sexual behavior includes	elevated ALT and
Healthcare worker with needle	multiple sexual partners, men	AST
stick injury or mucosal exposure to	having sex with men	HBV or HIV
HCV + blood		infection

Q. How to evaluate a patient with HCV Infection?
Ans: The approach to evaluation of a patient with HCV is elaborated below:
  Diagnosis of HCV infection:

- Anti-HCV

  Virological assessment:

- Quantitative HCV RNA
- HCV genotype (in selected cases)
- Resistance-associated substitutions (in selected cases)

  Assessment of liver disease severity:

- Noninvasive assessment of fibrosis—serum tests: APRI, FIB-4 and Transient Elastography (TE).
- Rule out cirrhosis based on TE >12.5 kPa, APRI, and FIB-4; if present, urgent treatment is warranted.
- Ancillary tests like USG/CT scan and AFP to rule out HCC.

  Evaluation for comorbidities/coinfections:

- Renal function tests
- HBsAg/HIV ELISA
- Pregnancy test in women of childbearing age

  Is HCV genotype testing mandatory before initiating DAA?
  Ans: With the availability of newer pan-genotypic DAA, the need for routine HCV genotype testing is not essential. However, genotype testing may be useful in:

- Selecting cost-effective therapies, especially in the setting of cirrhosis
- Predicting prognosis (worse with genotype 3 infection)
- Determining relapse vs reinfection

  What are the conditions in which urgent treatment may be initiated in HCV patients?

- Presence of advanced fibrosis or cirrhosis, including decompensated cirrhosis (depending upon CTP, MELD scores, eligibility, and expected time frame for transplantation).
- Extrahepatic manifestations (cryoglobulinemic vasculitis, HCV-associated nephropathy, and lymphoma).
- Recurrence of HCV post-liver transplant.
- Patients on immunosuppressive therapies, and those with HIV-HCV coinfection.
- Individuals at high risk of HCV transmission.

Q. What are the contraindications to HCV therapy?

The use of certain CYP/P enzyme inducers (such as carbamazepine, phenytoin, and phenobarbital) are contraindicated with all regimens due to the risk of significantly reduced concentrations DAAs and, therefore the high risk of virological failure.

Treatment regimens consists of an NS3-4A protease inhibitors, such as grazoprevir, glecaprevir, or voxilaprevir, are contraindicated in patients with decompensated (Child-Pugh B or C) cirrhosis and in patients with previous episodes of decompensation because of the substantially higher protease inhibitor concentrations in these patients and the increased risk of toxicity.

Q. How will you manage this patient in question?

Ans:

Confirmation of HCV infection (HCV RNA+)

- Baseline investigations: APRI, FIB-4, transient elastography (if available)
- In non-cirrhotic patients: Treat with Sofosbuvir (400 mg)+Daclatasvir (60 mg) × 12 weeks.
- Check HCV RNA after 12 weeks of treatment completion for sustained virological response (SVR).
- HCV RNA not detected: Treatment completed and SVR achieved.

Cirrhosis (Compensated Child-Pugh A)

- Treat with Sofosbuvir (400 mg) + Velpatasvir (100 mg) for 12 weeks.
- Check HCV RNA 12 weeks after treatment completion.
- HCV RNA not detected: Treatment completed.
- If HCV RNA detectable: Linkage pathway to a higher center for expert opinion and management.

Decompensated cirrhosis (Child-Pugh B/C)

- Sofosbuvir (400 mg) + Velpatasvir (100 mg) + Ribavirin (600–1200 mg) for 12 weeks.
- If Ribavirin intolerant/ineligible: Sofosbuvir (400 mg) + Velpatasvir (100 mg) for 24 weeks.

Treatment experienced with NS5A inhibitors

Sofosbuvir (400 mg) + Velpatasvir (100 mg) + Ribavirin (600–1200 mg) for 24 weeks.

AASLD 2019: Simplified treatment

Simplified treatment for chronic Hepatitis C (non-cirrhotic)

Non-eligibility criteria:

- Prior treatment
- ESRD (eGFR<30 ml/min/m^2)

- HIV/HBV coinfection
- Current pregnancy
- Known/suspected HCC
- Prior liver transplantation

Pre-treatment assessment:

(a) Pre-treatment laboratory testing
(b) Cirrhosis assessment: A patient is considered to have cirrhosis if any one of the following is present:
   1. FIB-4 score> 3.25
   2. TE>12.5 KPa
   3. Noninvasive serologic test above proprietary cut-offs for cirrhosis (Fibrotest, ELF test)
   4. Clinical evidence of cirrhosis (e.g., liver nodularity and/or splenomegaly on imaging)
   5. Prior documented cirrhosis on liver biopsy
(c) Potential drug–drug interaction assessment
(d) Education of patients

Recommended regimens:

- Glecaprevir 300 mg/Pibrentasvir 120 mg taken with food for eight weeks.
- Sofosbuvir 400 mg/Velpatasvir 100 mg for 12 weeks.

Simplified treatment for chronic Hepatitis C with compensated cirrhosis
Non-eligibility criteria: As mentioned before.
Pre-treatment assessment: As mentioned above.
Recommended regimens:

- Genotypes 1–6: Glecaprevir 300 mg/Pibrentasvir 120 mg taken with food for 8 weeks.
- Genotypes 1,2,4,5,6: Sofosbuvir 400 mg/Velpatasvir 100 mg for 12 weeks.
- *(Baseline NS5A RAS for genotype 3 is recommended.)*

Q. How should a patient be monitored on Ribavirin therapy?
Ans: Ribavirin can cause hemolysis and may rapidly lead to symptomatic anemia. If associated with symptoms, a reduction in hemoglobin (Hb) levels to 10 g/dl or less should trigger ribavirin dose reduction to 600 mg. If Hb drops to 8.5 g/dl or less, temporary discontinuation of ribavirin is advised. For patients with known ischemic heart disease, much closer monitoring is recommended, with reduction or discontinuation of therapy if Hb decreases by >2 g/dl compared to baseline. Hb should be tested periodically at 0, 2, 4, 6, 8, 10, 12 weeks. Closer monitoring (weekly) is indicated where Hb decline is rapid.

Other side effects of ribavirin are development of rash, shortness of breath, nausea, sore throat, cough, and glossitis. The rash may be severe and require ribavirin discontinuation. Ribavirin is teratogenic, so both men and women should be advised to practice effective contraception during therapy and for six months of treatment completion.

Q. What is the role of Resistance Associated Substitution (RAS) testing in the management of HCV?

Ans: Pre-treatment evaluation of RAS is indicated in specific situations depending upon the type of regimen used.

Sofosbuvir/Velpatasvir and Sofosbuvir/Daclatasvir

NS5A RAS Y93H is recommended for genotype 3 (AASLD 2019).

If present: Add Ribavirin or Voxilaprevir (contraindicated in decompensated cirrhosis as it is a protease inhibitor).

Elbasvir/Grazoprevir

In Genotype 1a: If RAS is present, an alternative regimen is advised.

Sofosbuvir/Ledipasvir

In genotype 1a, who are treatment-experienced and if NS5A RAS is present, alternative therapy should be considered.

EASL 2020: Testing for HCV resistance before first-line treatment is not recommended.

Q. How to follow up with patients in the post-treatment period?

Ans: The following key points need to be assessed during patient follow-up

Post-treatment assessment of cure (SVR)

Assessment of quantitative HCV RNA and hepatic function panel is recommended 12 weeks or later following completion of therapy to confirm virologic cure and normalization of transaminases.

Assessment for other causes of liver disease is recommended for patients with persistently elevated transaminase levels after achieving SVR.

Follow-up after achieving virologic cure

No liver-related follow up is currently recommended for non-cirrhotic patients who achieve SVR.

In non-cirrhotic patients with HCV who have achieved SVR after antiviral therapy, the American Gastroentrology Association (AGA) suggests a post-treatment TE cut-off of 9.5 kPa to rule out advanced liver fibrosis (AGA 2017).

Patients with ongoing risk for HCV infection (e.g., Intravenous drug users, males having sex with male engaging in unprotected sex) should be counselled about risk reduction and tested for HCV RNA annually and also when they develop elevated ALT, AST, or bilirubin.

In compensated cirrhosis

Post-treatment assessment of cure (SVR): Similar to non-cirrhotic cases.

Follow-up after achieving virologic cure:

American association for the study of the liver diseases (AASLD) guidelines recommend ultrasound surveillance for HCC (with or without AFP) every six months.

Upper GI endoscopy surveillance for esophageal varices is recommended according to AASLD guidelines for portal hypertensive bleeding in cirrhosis.

Abstinence from alcohol intake.

Patients with ongoing risk for HCV infection (e.g., IVDU, MSM engaging in unprotected sex) should be counseled about risk reduction and tested for HCV RNA annually and whenever they develop elevated ALT, AST, or bilirubin.

Q. How to manage HCV infection in special population groups?
Ans: DAA treatment in special situations.

(a) Decompensated cirrhosis:

Points to remember:

- Treat with caution:
  - The patient may worsen with treatment: Counsel patient and ensure close follow-up.
  - Drug toxicity
    Protease inhibitors are contraindicated
    Ribavirin may lead to severe anemia
- Add Ribavirin if not contraindicated, start with lower doses
- Keep MELD purgatory in mind
  - If MELD >18 and CTP-C, the risk may outweigh the benefits, and treatment may be considered after liver transplantation.

ELITA consensus statement on the use of DAA in LT candidates (Belli et al, JHepatol 2017)

- Overall, 20% of patients have an improvement in liver functions and can be de-listed.
- MELD <16: 35% may be delisted
- MELD 16–20: 12% may be delisted
- MELD 20–25: Minority may show improvement and be delisted
- MELD >25: DAA not recommended

International LT society consensus statement: (Terrault et al., Transplantation 2017)

- CTP B and/or MELD <20: DAA before transplant.

What are the pros and cons of HCV treatment in LT-eligible HCV cirrhosis?

Pros	Cons
Achieve reasonable SVR rate >80%	May lead to delisting from liver transplant due to improved MELD scores but yet continue to have a poor quality of life (MELD purgatory)
Improved hepatic function	Preclude the use of HCV-positive donor organs
May improve quality of life and liver-related complications in some patients	Patients are still at risk for HCC
Improved MELD and CTP scores which can lead to either inactivation or delisting from the liver transplant list (20–30%)	Treatment in patients with high MELD scores (MELD >20, CTP C) is associated with lower SVR rates and more adverse effects, and less likelihood of improvement in hepatic function
Reduced burden on LT waiting lists	
Prevent post-LT HCV recurrence	
Fewer drug–drug interactions compared to treating in the post-LT setting	
It may be the only option in patients who are not candidates for LT or where LT is not readily available	

(b) **Post-liver transplant:**

The natural course of HCV infection is accelerated post-LT; 15–30% of patients progress to cirrhosis within 5 years and 2–9% of patients may develop fibrosing cholestatic hepatitis (FCH).

Optimal timing for starting therapy: Soon after LT, once the immediate post-operative issues are resolved and before significant liver disease develops, stable immunosuppression levels are achieved, and with no ongoing episode of acute rejection.

Drug interactions need special consideration, especially protease inhibitors with calcineurin and mTOR inhibitors; NS5A inhibitors with everolimus. SOF/DCV, SOF/VEL can be given safely with most immunosuppression regimens.

AASLD recommendation post-LT management:
Glecaprevir (400 mg) + Pibrentasvir (120 mg) × 12 weeks
Sofosbuvir (400 mg) + Velpatasvir (100 mg) × 12 weeks
Sofosbuvir (400 mg) + Ledipasvir (90 mg) × 12 weeks (For Genotype 1,4,5,6)

(c) **CKD patients:**

The rationale for HCV therapy in patients with CKD:

• In patients in whom kidney transplant is not possible: HCV cure can reduce all-cause mortality.

- Curing HCV would lead to better graft and patient outcomes after a living donor renal transplant.
- Advanced fibrosis (F3) and compensated cirrhosis: HCV cure can potentially avoid the need for a liver transplant.
- Sofosbuvir combination therapy along with daclatasvir/ledipasvir/velpatasvir is safe and efficacious across various studies from India and abroad.
- No dose adjustments of directly acting antivirals are needed as per the AASLD.

(d) **Pregnancy:**

Chronic infection may develop in 3–5% of the babies in mothers with chronic HCV with an increased risk in HIV positive population.

Treatment before pregnancy: Ribavirin teratogenic (both males and females).

Treatment during pregnancy: Not recommended at this stage (Preliminary studies have shown safety in pregnancy with Sofosbuvir–Ledipasvir in HCV genotype 1, *Chappell et al., Lancet, 2020*).

Delivery: Avoid invasive procedures like fetal scalp monitors, instrument-assisted delivery, etc.

After delivery: Breastfeeding is not contraindicated unless there is the presence of cracked nipple. A spontaneous clearance occurs in 10–25% in the post-partum period. It is optimal to wait for 9–12 months post-partum to initiate DAAs.

Evaluation of child: Anti-HCV at 18 months, if positive-HCV RNA at three years.

(e) **Children:**

Treat at or more than 3 years of age.

Early antiviral treatment is indicated if there is the presence of advanced fibrosis or extrahepatic manifestations like cryoglobulinemia, rash, or glomerulonephritis.

AASLD recommendation:

>12 years or weight >45 kg: Glecaprevir/Pibrentasvir × 8 weeks

Age > 3years, GT (genotype) 1,4,5,6: Sofosbuvir/Ledipasvir × 12 weeks

Dose: Sof: <17 kg–150 mg; 17–35 kg–200 mg; >35 kg: 400 mg

Ledipasvir: <17 kg–33.75 mg; 17–35 kg: 45 mg; >35 kg: 90 mg

Age 3–11 years: GT 2,3: Sofosbuvir + Ribavirin

Dose: Ribavirin: <47 kg: 15 mg/kg

(f) **HIV/HCV coinfection:**

Important drug interactions and points:

- Daclatasvir requires a reduction in dose with boosted PI regimens like ritonavir–atazanavir (reduce to 30 mg/day) and increased dosage with regimens containing efavirenz or etravirine (increase to 90 mg/day).
- Fixed-dose combination (FDC) of Sofosbuvir-Velpatasvir cannot be used with efavirenz, etravirine, or nevirapine.

- Both FDC of Sofosbuvir–Velpatasvir and Sof–Ledi increase tenofovir (TDF) level when TDF is used and should be avoided in patients with eGFR <60 ml/min. Tenofovir alefenamide may be an alternative.
- Ribavirin should not be used with didanosine, stavudine, or zidovudine due to the risk of rapidly worsening anemia and risk of pancreatitis.
- Interruption of ART (anti-retroviral therapy) to allow HCV therapy is not indicated.
- Anti-HCV can be false negative in HIV patients with low CD4, and the presence of HCV infection may need to be confirmed by quantitative HCV RNA.
- SVR rate is comparable to mono-infected patients.

HBV/HCV coinfection:

	AASLD	EASL
HBsAg+ve Non-cirrhotic	Risk of flare during DAA treatment During therapy, monitor HBV DNA, ALT q4-8 weeks and for 3 months post-treatment	Recommends concomitant NA prophylaxis until week 12 post-DAA therapy
HBsAg-ve, Anti-HBc +ve	Low risk of flares during DAA Monitor ALT at baseline, during follow-up and end of treatment If ALT increases, or does not normalize during therapy or post-therapy, then monitor HBsAg and HBV DNA	Test for HBV reactivation in case of raised ALT levels

Q. How is a diagnosis of acute HCV infection made, and what are the recommended treatment options?

An acute HCV infection should be suspected in an appropriate clinical setting which involves a high risk of acquiring an HCV infection (PWIDs, hemodialysis patients, patients on repeated blood transfusions, recent needlestick injury, incarcerated population, etc.).

The confirmatory evidence of diagnosing acute HCV is classically seen in two circumstances:

- A positive HCV antibody test after a documented prior negative HCV antibody test (seroconversion).
- A positive HCV RNA test in the setting of a negative HCV antibody test (identification during the seronegative window period).

In patients who do not have a definitive history of exposure and in whom baseline HCV antibody test is unavailable, diagnosis can be difficult. Such patients should be suspected if there is a rising ALT level without an alternate cause or there is a low (especially <104 IU/mL) or fluctuating (>1 $\log_{10}$ IU/mL) HCV RNA level.

HCV clears spontaneously in 20–50% of such patients. However, according to the recent AASLD guidelines (2019), HCV treatment should be initiated in acute HCV without waiting for spontaneous clearance because of:

1. High efficacy and safety of currently available DAA therapy.
2. Risk of loss to subsequent follow-up.
3. Decrease risk of transmission of HCV.

Q. What is occult HCV infection?

Occult HCV infection is a rarely encountered situation of undetermined clinical significance where HCV RNA can be detected in liver tissue either alone or in both liver tissue and peripheral blood mononuclear cells (PBMCs) with persistently undetectable serum HCV RNA levels. This can be seen in two phenotypic profiles:

*   Detectable HCV RNA in liver tissue of patients being evaluated for unknown liver disease (anti-HCV negative, serum HCV RNA negative, liver tissue HCV RNA +).
*   Detectable HCV RNA in liver tissue of patients with spontaneous/post-treatment clearance of HCV (anti-HCV +, serum HCV RNA negative, liver tissue HCV RNA +).

Further Readings

Ghany MG, et al. AASLD-IDSA recommendations for testing, managing, and treating hepatitis C virus infection. Hepatology. 2020;71(2):686–721.

National Guidelines for Diagnosis & Management of Viral Hepatitis. https://www.inasl.org.in/diagnosis-management-viral-hepatitis.pdf

Non-alcoholic Fatty Liver Disease (NAFLD)

5

Ajay Duseja, Akash Roy, and Virendra Singh

Case Vignette A 44-year gentleman presented to the outpatient department after being referred for elevated liver enzymes during a routine annual check-up. He had no history of alcohol intake but was hypertensive and had type 2 diabetes mellitus (T2DM) and was on Metformin hydrochloride and Olmesartan 20. He has a family history of coronary artery disease, dyslipidemia, and T2DM. He is an engineer by occupation consuming a mixed diet and has a sedentary lifestyle. Height and body weight were 168 cm and 88 kg, respectively, with a body mass index (BMI) of 31.2 kg/m^2 and a waist circumference of 92 cm. On examination, he had a BP of 144/87 mmHg and pulse rate of 72/min. Systemic examination was unremarkable.

Laboratory investigations revealed the following:

Parameter	Values	Parameter	Values
Hemoglobin	11	INR	1
Platelet count	140	HBsAg	Non-reactive
Total leukocyte count	7000	Anti HCV	Neg
Total bilirubin (Direct)	1(0.8)	HbA$_1$C	6.7
AST	44	S Na/K	130/4.3
ALT	56	Albumin	3.6
ALP	89	Urea/ Creatinine	40/1
Lipid profile (Triglyceride/Low density lipoprotein/High density lipoprotein)	265/78/20	Urine routine	Albumin 1+, Rest normal

USG W/A: Liver 12 cm, bright echotexture normal in outline. Portal vein—Normal. Spleen 8 cm. No free fluid

A. Duseja · A. Roy · V. Singh (✉)
Department of Hepatology, Post Graduate Institute of Medical Education and Research, Chandigarh, Punjab, India

35

How Is NAFLD diagnosed? What are the definitions for NAFL and NASH?

The diagnosis of NAFLD depends on two essential characteristics which include:

- Demonstration of the presence of fat (steatosis) in the liver either by any imaging modality or on evaluation of histology in biopsy specimen.
- Absence of secondary causes of fat accumulation (significant alcohol consumption, prolonged medication use proven to cause hepatic steatosis or hereditary disorders associated with fat accumulation).

NAFLD exists in two predominant forms—NAFL (non-alcoholic fatty liver) and NASH (non-alcoholic steatohepatitis). NAFL is defined as the presence of steatotic changes in liver of more than 5% without evidence of hepatocellular injury. NASH is defined as the presence NAFL along with inflammation with hepatocyte injury with or without fibrosis.

Q. What Are the Established and Evolving Risk Factors for NAFLD?

Presence of metabolic syndrome (MetS) both as a composite entity as well as individual components of MetS forms the strongest risk factors for NAFLD. The risk factors can be classified as those that are established and few that are evolving as potential risk factors (Table 5.1).

Q. Describe in brief the association of Metabolic Syndrome and its components with NAFLD

NAFLD and MetS are intrinsically interlinked with a bidirectional association. On one hand, individual components of MetS are seen with a high prevalence in patients with NAFLD, whereas on the other hand presence of MetS components are associated with an increased risk of developing NAFLD. Greater than 90% of patients with NAFLD have at least one feature of MetS and up to one-third have all the components. High BMI and presence of visceral obesity have been shown to be the most important predictors of NAFLD with European literature suggesting that 65–90% of NAFLD patients being overweight or obese (Chowdhury A, Younossi

Table 5.1 Risk factors for NAFLD

Established risk factors	Evolving risk factors
Metabolic syndrome	Obstructive sleep apnea
Obesity	Endocrinopathies
Type II diabetes	Polycystic ovarian disease not related to obesity
Dyslipidemia	Psoriasis
Hypertension	Osteoporosis
Age	Colorectal cancer
Controversial: Sex, ethnicity	

2016). Literature from bariatric surgery suggests that 95% of people who are severely obese have NAFLD (Subichin et al. 2015). One study has shown that diabetics have 4 times more risk of having NAFLD 9OR, 4.16; (95% CI, 3.24–5.33) (Zebb et al 2013). Furthermore, the severity of NAFLD and its progression to NASH is proportional to the number of metabolic risk factors. Zebb et al. have shown that the chances of developing NAFLD when three components of MetS are present is 9.49 (95 % CI, 5.67 five components are present, the odds increase to 24.05 (95 % CI, 12.73–45.45).

Q. What are the mechanisms involved in Hepatic Steatosis and development of NAFLD?
The key biochemical alterations that lead to increased steatosis include:

- Increased free fatty acid flux (FFA) from the adipocytes to hepatocytes
- Increased hepatic uptake of FFA from the circulation
- Insulin-mediated stimulation of hepatic lipogenesis
- Glucose-mediated stimulation of hepatic lipogenesis
- Endoplasmic reticulum (ER) stress-mediated stimulation of hepatic lipogenesis
- ER stress-mediated inhibition of hepatic lipid export

The key alterations are schematically shown in Fig. 5.1.

Q. Mention the Noninvasive Measures for Assessment of Fibrosis in NAFLD (Table 5.2)

Q. What are the elastography-based tests used in the assessment of fibrosis in NAFLD?
Transient Elastography (Fibroscan): Transient elastography (with M probe and XL probe, especially in obese patients) has become a widely available tool for measuring liver stiffness. It is based on vibration controlled elastography (VCTE) technique which estimates the degree of liver "stiffness," as a function of the extent of hepatic fibrosis. Using validated cut-offs 7–10 kPa the technique has fair accuracy for ruling out and ruling in advanced fibrosis, respectively. Additionally, at a cut-off of 5.9 kPa it has a sensitivity of 86.1% and specificity of 88.9% for detection of fibrosis.

Acoustic radiation force impulse imaging (ARFI): It is based on the principle of a focused shear wave to generate B-mode ultrasound image. The system can be integrated as a part of conventional ultrasonography systems to assess fibrosis. Units are provided in m/sec. Its principal advantages include that it is not affected by the presence of obesity or ascites. However, it has a poor discriminatory value for intermediate-stage fibrosis.

MR Elastography: Its principal advantage lies in the fact that it can assess the entire liver and is not affected by obesity and ascites. However, cannot be used in iron-overload states. It has a sensitivity of 85% and specificity of 93% using a cut-off 4.15 kPa for the diagnosis of advanced fibrosis (AUROC 0.95).

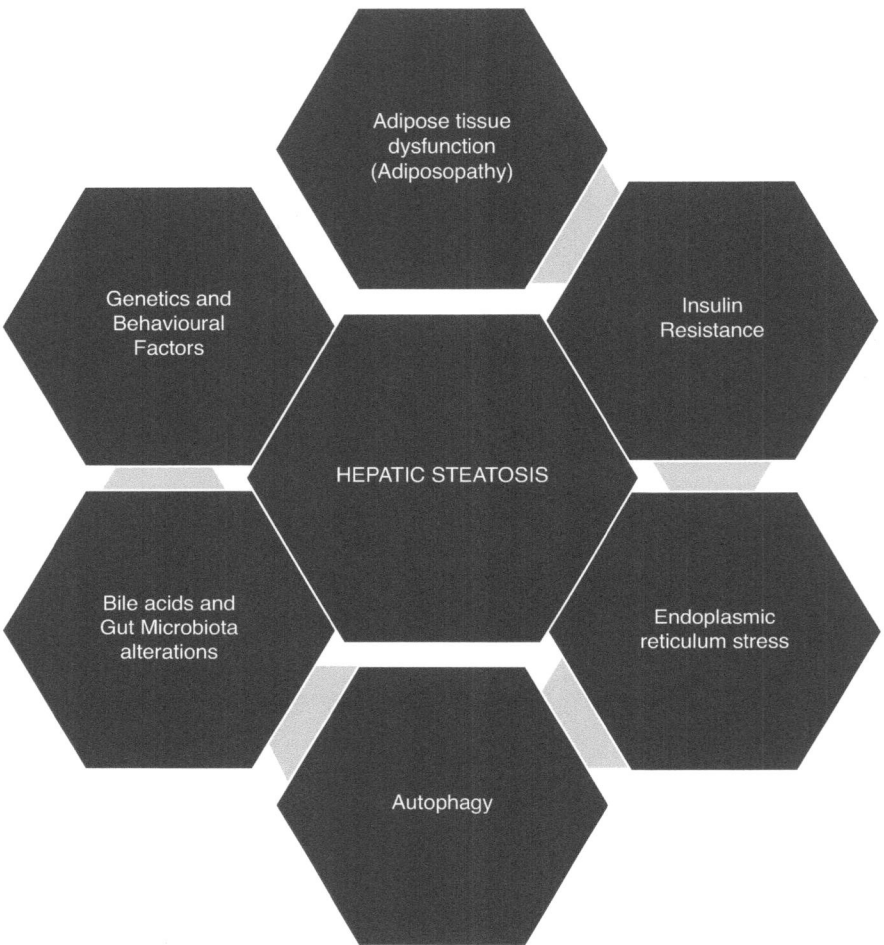

Fig. 5.1 Mechanisms leading to hepatic steatosis

Table 5.2 Noninvasive measures for fibrosis assessment in NAFLD

Serum-based tests	Components	AUROC	Specificity/Sensitivity (%)
APRI	AST, platelet count	0.80	89/27
Fib-4	Age, AST, platelet, ALT	0.86	26/98 (at 3.25 cut off)
NAFLD fibrosis score	Age, BMI, hyperglycemia, platelet, albumin, AST/ALT ratio	0.81	98/33(at 0.676)
Enhanced Liver Fibrosis (ELF) test	Age, HA, TIMP-1, PIIINP	0.82–0.9	90/80

APRI AST Platelet Ratio Index, *Fib-4* Fibrosis-4, *AST* Aspartate transaminase, *ALT* Alanine transaminase, *BMI* Body mass index, *HA* Hyaluronic acid, *TIMP* Tissue inhibitors of metalloproteinases, Procollagen III N-Terminal Propeptide, *AUROC* Area under receiving operating curve, **Sp* Specificity, **Sn* Sensitivity

Q. What are the risks of Hepatocellular Carcinoma (HCC) associated with NAFLD?

NAFLD has been shown to be one of the fastest growing causes for HCC, which is driven in part by the overall high prevalence of NAFLD. The overall estimated annual incidence of HCC among patients with NAFLD cirrhosis ranges from 0.5% to 2.6%, which is partly lower than viral hepatitis (Huang DQ et al. Nature Reviews Gastroenterology & Hepatology. 2021). However, the sheer magnitude of NAFLD makes NAFLD-related HCC one of the fastest growing diseases of concern. Another, unique aspect of NAFLD and HCC is the presence of non-cirrhotic HCC in NAFLD (incidence 1.3/1000 patient-years). The evolution of HCC in patients with NAFLD without evidence of cirrhosis has been widely established and may occur in about 30–50% of patients. On comparison of non-cirrhotic patients with NAFLD with or without HCC, some key factors that have been associated with an increased risk of HCC include: male gender, light drinker, and high Fibrosis-4 index (Tobari M et al. JGH 2020).

Q. Outline the principles of management of NAFLD

The principles of NAFLD management include:
  Weight loss measures:

- Definitive evidence exists regarding the impact of weight loss in NAFLD. In a landmark study, it was shown that achieving a weight loss of ≥7% led to significant improvements in all features of liver histology (Pomrat et al. Hepatology 2010). Furthermore, weight loss of ≥10% leads to improvement of fibrosis (Glass et al Dig Ds Sci 2015).

Lifestyle modifications:

- **Restriction of caloric intake:** 1200–1600 calories restricted diet with preferable consumption of a Mediterranean diet. In a comparative study of the Mediterranean diet with low-fat, high-carbohydrate diet, a histological improvement of steatosis with Mediterranean diet has been reported (Tendler et al Dig Ds Sc 2007).
- **Physical Exercise:** Kistler et al. showed that an exercise regimen for 75 min/week leads to improvement of NASH histology (Kistler et al Am J Gastro 2011). However, emerging evidence suggests that overall, 150–200 min every week of aerobic and resistance training is optimal.

Pharmacotherapeutics
Vitamin E:

- Acts primarily as an antioxidant.
- **PIVENS Trial** (Sanyal et al NEJM 2010): 247 NASH patients without DM were assigned in a 3-arm trial to receive pioglitazone (30 mg daily), vitamin E (800 IU daily), or placebo for 96 weeks. The primary outcome was an improvement in NASH histology. Vitamin E led to significant improvement in steatosis, hepatic

transaminase levels, steatohepatitis, and histology as compared to placebo. However, there were no significant changes in fibrosis.

- It may be considered in non-diabetic patients with NASH, although concerns remain about all-cause mortality, hemorrhagic stroke, and risk of prostate cancer.
- In another recent study, the use of Vitamin E has been associated with an improved clinical outcome in patients with NASH who have bridging fibrosis or compensated cirrhosis (Vilar Gomez Hepatology 2018).

Pioglitazone
It is a Peroxisome proliferator-activated receptor gamma (PPAR-γ) agonist established as an antidiabetic medication. It has been found to reduce steatosis, hepatic transaminase, and also leads to an improvement in histology. However, concerns remain about weight gain, risk of bladder cancer, and an unsubstantiated cardiac risk (Sanyal et al NEJM 2010).

Obeticholic acid (OCA)
OCA is an Farnesoid X receptor agonist. Two landmark trials namely the FLINT trial and the REGENERATE trial have shown the efficacy of OCA in NASH. The FLINT trial was a phase 2 placebo-controlled trial that showed improvement in histologic markers of NASH with treatment with OCA 25 mg daily (Neuschwander et al. Lancet 2015). The results of the 18-month interim analysis of the REGENERATE trial showed that OCA at a dose of 25 mg daily led to improvement of fibrosis without worsening of NASH in 21.0% ($p<0.001$) and resolution of NASH without worsening of fibrosis in 14.9% ($p = 0.001$) (Younossi et al Lancet 2019).

Emerging therapies in NASH: Multiple emerging therapies are in various phases of clinical trials in NASH. However, some of the promising agents are shown in Table 5.3.

Q. What is meant by the term MAFLD?
The term "MAFLD" is a recently introduced term to provide a more holistic approach to the diagnosis of liver steatosis arising out of metabolic dysfunction and stands for "Metabolic dysfunction associated fatty liver disease." The proposed criteria for MAFLD are based on evidence of hepatic steatosis on histology (biopsy), imaging, or blood biomarker evidence in addition to one of the following three

Table 5.3 Emerging drug therapies in NASH

Drug	Mechanism of action	Trial
Elafibrinor	PPARα/δ agonist	GOLDEN-505 trial
Semaglutide	GLP-1mimetic	
Cenicriviroc	CCR2 CCR5 inhibitor	CENTAUR trial
Saroglitazor	PPARα/Υ agonist	EVIDENCES trial
Selenosertib	ASK1 inhibitor	Negative results with initial trial
Resmetirom	THR-β agonist	MAESTRO-NASH trial

criteria, namely overweight/obesity, presence of type 2 diabetes mellitus (T2DM), or evidence of metabolic dysregulation. Metabolic dysregulation is in turn defined as presence of at least two of the following criteria:

- Waist circumference ≥102/88 cm in Caucasian men and women or ≥90/80 cm in Asian men and women.
- Blood pressure ≥130/85 mmHg or specific drug treatment.
- Plasma triglycerides ≥150 mg/dL (≥1.70 mmol/l) or specific drug treatment.
- Plasma HDL-cholesterol <40 mg/dL (<1.0 mmol/L) for men and <50 mg/dL (<1.3 mmol/L) for women or specific drug treatment.
- Prediabetes (i.e., fasting glucose levels 100–125 mg/dL (5.6–6.9 mmol/L), or 2-h post-load glucose levels 140–199 mg/dL (7.8–11.0 mmol) or HbA1c 5.7–6.4% (39–47 mmol/mol)).
- Homeostasis model assessment (HOMA)-insulin resistance score ≥2.5.
- Plasma high-sensitivity C-reactive protein (hs-CRP) level >2 mg/L.

Further Reading

Friedman SL, et al. Mechanisms of NAFLD development and therapeutic strategies. Nat Med. 2018;24(7):908–22.
Duseja A, et al. Epidemiology and risk factors of nonalcoholic fatty liver disease (NAFLD). Hepatol Int. 2013;7(Suppl 2):755–64.

Alcoholic Hepatitis

6

Nipun Verma, Akash Roy, and Virendra Singh

Case Vignette

A 42-year-old male software engineer presents with a two-week history of progressive non-cholestatic jaundice. He has no history of any background medical comorbidities or any history of major surgical intervention. There is no history of any chronic drug intake or history of complementary and alternative medicine intake. He consumes 40–60 gm of whiskey five times a week for the last 5 years with a tendency to have increased drinks over the weekends. Over the last 1 month, his alcohol consumption has increased significantly on account of job-related stress and consumes 100–120 gm of alcohol daily. He is a nonsmoker, has no other addictions, and has never had any tattoos, blood transfusion, or unsafe needle practices. He has a BMI of 24 kg/m². He is afebrile and has a BP 100/60 mm Hg, PR 110/min, and RR 16/min. His physical exam is remarkable for scleral icterus, multiple spider angiomas, and the presence of palmar erythema. Per abdominal examination is remarkable for an enlarged firm liver (span of 16 cm) and a palpable spleen. There is no free fluid in the abdomen.

Laboratory investigations revealed the following:

Parameter	Values	Parameter	Values
Hemoglobin	10.2	INR	1.6
Platelet count	120	HBsAg	NR
Total leukocyte count	12,000	Anti-HCV	Neg
Total bilirubin (Direct)	8 (5.3)	ANA/ASMA	Negative
AST	144	S Na/K	132/4.3
ALT	62	Urea	32
ALP	91	Creatinine	1
Albumin	3.2	Ig M HAV/HEV	Negative

N. Verma · A. Roy · V. Singh (✉)
Department of Hepatology, Post Graduate Institute of Medical Education and Research, Chandigarh, Punjab, India

© The Author(s), under exclusive license to Springer Nature Singapore Pte Ltd. 2022
V. Singh, A. Roy (eds.), *Clinical Rounds in Hepatology*, https://doi.org/10.1007/978-981-16-8448-7_6

An abdominal ultrasound was done, which showed an enlarged liver with coarse echotexture and an enlarged spleen. The gallbladder and biliary system were unremarkable. Portal vein diameter was 13 mm, and there was no free fluid.

Q1. What Is the most probable diagnosis based on the given Vignette?
Ans: Alcoholic Hepatitis.

Q. How Is the Diagnosis of Alcoholic Hepatitis (AH) made?
AH is a classic clinical presentation that has the hallmark of an abrupt development of jaundice in a setting of heavy antecedent alcohol use. Recent heavy alcohol consumption is a cardinal feature in the history of AH. To arrive at a consensus for uniformity of definitions, the **NIAAA (National Institute on Alcohol Abuse and Alcoholism)** established the following standard definitions:

Minimum criteria for diagnosis	Possible alcoholic hepatitis
• Serum bilirubin >3.0 mg/dL. • Consumption of more than 3 standard drinks (40 grams) per day for females and 4 drinks (50–60 grams) per day for males for greater than 6 months. • Less than 60 days from last drink to the development of jaundice. • AST >50 IU/L but AST and ALT less than 400 IU/L. • AST:ALT ratio of >1.5.	Does not meet minimum criteria OR has potential confounders • Inconsistent alcohol history. • Atypical laboratory studies (AST < 50, ALT/AST > 400, or AST:ALT ratio < 1.5). • Recent shock (hemorrhagic or septic). • Positive immune markers (ANA >1:160 or ASMA >1:80). • Possibility of DILI. *Liver Biopsy is recommended to confirm diagnosis*
Probable alcoholic hepatitis: Meets minimum criteria for AH without confounding factors Negative immune markers (ANA <1:160, ASMA <1:80 dilution) Absence of sepsis, shock, cocaine use, or drug use at risk of DILI within 30 days *Liver biopsy is not mandatory for diagnosis*	**Definite alcoholic hepatitis:** Clinical AH and biopsy-proven AH

Q. What percentage of heavy drinkers develop cirrhosis?
10% to 20% of those who chronically use at least 50 g of alcohol daily for more than 5 years will develop cirrhosis.

Q. Do all patients with AH have cirrhosis?
Around 80% of patients presenting with AH will have underlying cirrhosis.

Q. What are the classical clinical features of AH?
The cardinal clinical symptom is jaundice. However, AH as a syndrome can have a various range of presentations, including mild hepatic derangements to frank signs of liver cell failure. Certain nonspecific symptoms include fever and/or leukocytosis, nausea, and anorexia. Right upper quadrant pain may be present, which is typically dull aching, and constant and occurs due to an enlarged liver causing stretching of the hepatic capsule. In cases of severe AH, there may be presence of ascites, variceal GI Bleed, cutaneous markers of coagulation failure, hepatic encephalopathy, and acute kidney injury.
Clinical findings:

- Features of SIRS (Systemic Inflammatory Response Syndrome) in the absence of infection.
- Spider angiomata, parotid enlargement (bilateral), palmar erythema.
- Tender hepatomegaly.
- Hepatic bruit.
- Splenomegaly (mild to moderate).
- Tachycardia and a systolic flow murmur.
- Ascites.

Q. What are the histological features of Alcoholic Hepatitis?
Alcohol-related liver disease may present with a wide variety of histological forms. These include simple hepatic steatosis, inflammatory steatohepatitis, fibrosis, and cirrhosis. Alcoholic Steatohepatitis (ASH) is one of the histological forms which is commonly seen in those presenting with the clinical syndrome of AH. However, it is important to note that although most patients with AH will have ASH, there are patients with AH whose histology may have only cirrhosis or other histologic varieties. The cardinal features of ASH on histology are macrovesicular steatosis, lobular neutrophilic infiltrate, Mallory-Denk bodies, satellitosis, megamitochondria, and chicken wire fibrosis.

Bonus points

Alcoholic foamy degeneration: Foamy fatty change in perivenular hepatocytes with massive cell swelling, bile pigment deposition in the cytoplasm, and a non-displaced nucleus Megamitochondria are also frequently seen.

Alcoholic fatty liver with cholestasis: Severe steatosis and marked cholestasis with minimal hepatic fibrosis.

Walking AH: Patients with histologic ASH but clinically asymptomatic and having only deranged aminotransferases.

Q. What is the Alcoholic Hepatitis Histology Score (AHHS)?

It is a prediction model to assess severity based upon histology originally developed in a Spanish cohort of 121 patients. It grades the severity into 3 stages (mild, intermediate, and severe) based on 4 histologic components, which include:

- Stage of fibrosis.
- Bilirubinostasis.
- Megamitochondria.
- PMN infiltration.

Q. What are the clinical scores to assess the severity of this patient?

It is important to assess the severity of patients with AH as those with severe AH have high short-term mortality. Multiple clinical scoring systems have been used and validated to grade the severity of AH.

Severity scores in AH	Components/ Formula	Cut off for severe AH
Maddrey discriminant function (mDF)	$4.6 \times$ [patient's PT− Control PT] + total bilirubin (mg/dL)	≥ 32
MELD	Total bilirubin, INR, creatinine	≥ 20 (not well defined)
Glasgow alcoholic Hepatitis score (GAHS)	Age, WBC count, urea, INR, bilirubin	≥ 9
ABIC	Age, bilirubin, INR, creatinine	> 9

Q. What is Lille Model?

Patients with severe AH are candidates for intervention therapies, the most commonly used are corticosteroids. The Lille Model is a dynamic model to assess favorable response to therapy in patients with severe AH treated with corticosteroids. The model includes patient age, total serum bilirubin, INR, albumin, and PT at the initiation of corticosteroids and then the total serum bilirubin on day 7 of treatment. A score of >0.45 after 7 days of corticosteroids predicts a low 6-month survival (25% vs. 85%) and are considered as non-responders to corticosteroids.

Bonus Points

Lille Model: Louvet A et al. The Lille model: a new tool for therapeutic strategy in patients with severe alcoholic hepatitis treated with steroids. Hepatology, 2007

Aim

- To generate a specific prognostic model to enable clinicians to identify subjects early on who are unlikely to survive.
- To propose new management based on this model.

Primary endpoint—6-month survival

Inclusion Criteria—All patients with a DF ≥ 32 or encephalopathy at admission were treated with corticosteroids if they fulfilled the following criteria:

- History of alcoholism.
- Biochemistry suggestive of alcoholic hepatitis.
- Absence of uncontrolled infection or recent GI hemorrhage (<15 days).
- TJLB.

Exclusion Criteria—Excluded patients with active peptic ulcers, neoplasms, HBsAg+, HIV.

Treatment Protocol—40 mg prednisolone is given daily for 28 days. Patients who were unable to take oral medicines were given 32 mg iv methylprednisolone.

Exploratory Cohort—320 patients were included from July 1990 to October 2001 in Beaujon, Beclere, and Saint-Antoine Hospitals and from October 2001 to October 2003 in the Lille Hospital.

Validating Cohort—Performed from November 2003 to April 2005 in 118 patients.

Results:

- **Baseline Characteristics ($n = 295$).**
  - Median age: 49.7 years.
  - Ascites: 78%.
  - Encephalopathy: 26.6%.
  - Median bilirubin (umol/l): 210 (32–877).
  - Prothrombin time: 19.5 (13.5–32).
  - White blood cell count: 10800 (2200–64,000).
  - Child Turcotte Pugh Score: 10 (7–15).
  - mDF: 47.5 (23.2–144.6).
- **Survival.**
  - 1 month: 86.5% ± 2%
  - 2 months: 77% ± 2.5%
  - 6 month: 65.4% ± 2.9%
- **Development of Lille Model.**
  - Final regression analysis yielded 6 variables—age, albumin at day 0, change in bilirubin levels, renal insufficiency, bilirubin at day 0, and PT in seconds (AUROC:0.89).
- **Management based on the Lille model.**
  - A value of 0.45 was determined for the highest predictive capacity (sensitivity and specificity of 76% and 85%, respectively, for overall population).
  - Patients with Lille score ≥ 0.45 had a significantly reduced 6-month survival (25 ± 3.8% vs. 85 ± 2.5%, $p < 0.01$).
  - In patients with a Lille score ≥ 0.45, there was no significant survival difference in 6-month survival between corticosteroid and placebo groups (27.8 ± 1% vs. 25.7 ± 7. %).
- **Limitations.**
  - Twenty-five percent of patients with a Lille score ≥ 0.45 did not die at 6 months; thus they are not true non-responders.
  - However, 50% of patients who were alive at 6 months had severe liver insufficiency with a median CTP of 8.5 (6–14) and a median MELD score of 21.5 (12–31).

Q. What are the management options for this patient?
General Measures

- Alcohol abstinence with careful assessment for alcohol withdrawal and its management.
- Nutritional support.
- Thiamine.
- Zinc supplementation.
- Surveillance for infections.

Specific measures

Corticosteroids: Standard international guidelines recommend a trial of 40 mg of prednisolone for 28 days in patients with severe AH. The basis of the recommendation is primarily derived from the largest randomized control trial known as the STOPAH (steroids or pentoxifylline for alcoholic hepatitis). In addition to the STOPAH trial, meta-analysis data of 2111 patients have shown that corticosteroid use is associated with a decreased risk of 28-day mortality. However, the overall benefit with corticosteroid therapy is modest, and the risks of therapy, including GI bleed, renal dysfunction, and most importantly, infections, need to be weighed prior to corticosteroid therapy.

Bonus points: STOPAH Trial
Thurz MR et al. NEJM 2015

Type of study; Multicentric double-blind randomized trial
Inclusion criteria: Clinical AH with an MDF of >32
Exclusion criteria: Creatinine >5.7 mg/dl, renal replacement therapy, uncontrolled sepsis, GI Bleed
Patients included: 1103
Key results:
Nonsignificant survival benefit at 28 days with prednisolone compared to placebo (OR 0.72; 95% CI, 0.52–1.01; $P = 0.06$).
Importantly on a post hoc multivariable analysis, prednisolone led to a decreased 28-day mortality (OR 0.609, $P = 0.015$), but not at 90 days or 1 year.

N-acetyl cysteine: NAC, when used along with corticosteroids, has been shown to provide a short-term (4–8 weeks) survival benefit but without any improvement in 6-month mortality.

Q. What are the options for Severe AH beyond corticosteroids?

Multiple investigational therapies are emerging in the management of severe AH, which include:

(Singal AK et al. Journal of Hepatology 2019)

- Granulocyte colony-stimulating factor (G-CSF).
- Fecal microbiota transplantation (FMT).
- Amoxycillin+Clavulinic acid.
- Metadoxine.
- Interleukin-22.

- Anakinra (IL-1 receptor antagonist).
- Obeticholic acid.
- Molecular adsorbent recycling system (MARS).

Q. What Is the current role of Pentoxifylline in the management of Severe AH?

Based upon the results of multiple RCTs as well as the STOPAH trial use of Pentoxifylline has no benefit in patients with AH. Pentoxifylline alone or even a combination of corticosteroids and Pentoxifylline offers no benefit (Louvet A et al. Gastroenterology. 2018).

Q. Give a brief review of the evidence for use of GCSF in AH

GCSF has been used in multiple studies with varying results. A summary of the available evidence is shown in table below.

Author/Year/ Location	Population	Arms	Number of patients	Dose of GCSF	90-day mortality
Spahr et al./2008/ Europe	AH	GCSF vs SOC	13 vs 11	10 ucg/kg/ day × 5 days	7.7% vs 0%
Garg et al./2012/ India	AH-ACLF	GCSF vs SOC	23 vs 24	5 ucg/ kg/d × 5 d and every 3 d for 1 month	30.4% vs 70.8%
Singh et al./2014/ India	Severe AH	GCSF + pentoxifylline vs pentoxifylline	23 vs 23	10 ucg/ kg/d × 5 d	21.7% vs 78%
Singh et al./2018/ India	Severe AH	SMT + GCSF+NAC vs SMT + GCSF+ vs SMT alone	19 vs 18 vs 20	10 ucg/ kg/d × 5 d	31% vs 11%vs 70%
Shastry et al./2019/ India	Severe AH who were steroid non-responders	GCSF vs placebo	14 vs 14	5ucg/kg/d × 5 d and every 3d × 1 month	35.7% vs 71.4%
Engelman et al./2019/ Europe	AH-ACLF	GCSF vs placebo	81 vs 82	5 ucg/ kg/d × 5 d and every 3 d × 1 month	66.7% vs 51.9%

Evidence from Marot A et al. JHEP Reports. 2020; *NAC* N-acetyl cysteine, *SMT* Standard medical therapy, *SOC* Standard of care

Q. What Is the Current Evidence for the Use of Fecal Microbiota Transplant (FMT) in Severe Alcoholic Hepatitis?

FMT has been used in small studies and has shown a potential benefit. In a study of 51 patients with 16 receiving FMT, 17 on only nutritional support, 8 receiving corticosteroids, and 10 receiving Pentoxifylline, FMT was shown to offer the maximum survival benefit (Philips CA et al. IJG 2018).

Further Reading

Singal AK, et al. Grand rounds: alcoholic hepatitis. J Hep. 2018;69(2):534–43.

Sehrawat TS, Liu M, Shah VH. The knowns and unknowns of treatment for alcoholic hepatitis. Lancet Gastroenterol Hepatol. 2020 May 1;5(5):494–506.

Acute on Chronic Liver Failure

7

Madhumita Premkumar, Akash Roy, and Virendra Singh

Case Vignette

A 32-year-old male, an alcohol consumer (150 gm/day × 5 years), and recent history of binge alcohol intake now presents with progressive jaundice for one month followed by abdominal distension for 15 days. There are no other significant medical comorbidities. There is no history suggestive of decreased urine output, shortness of breath, gastrointestinal bleed, or alteration in sensorium. On examination, he is deeply icteric and has parotid enlargement with bilateral pedal edema. Per abdominal examination is remarkable for an enlarged firm irregular liver and presence of ascites.

Laboratory investigations revealed the following:

Parameter	Values	Parameter	Values
Hemoglobin	10.2	INR	1.8
Platelet count	120	HBsAg	NR
Total leukocyte count	14,000	Anti-HCV	Neg
Total bilirubin (Direct)	10(6.5)	ANA/ASMA	Negative
AST	144	S Na/K	129/4.3
ALT	62	Urea	55
ALP	91	Creatinine	1.3 ˙
Albumin	3.2	Ig M HAV/ HEV (Hepatitis A, Hepatitis E)	Negative

Ascitic fluid analysis: Cells 200 N 60% L40%, Protein 1.8, Sugar 67, SAAG 1.3

USG abdomen: Liver (16 cm) with coarse echotexture and an enlarged spleen. The gallbladder and biliary system were unremarkable. Portal vein diameter was 13 mm with moderate ascites. Spleen 12 cm.

M. Premkumar · A. Roy · V. Singh (✉)
Department of Hepatology, Post Graduate Institute of Medical Education and Research, Chandigarh, Punjab, India

V. Singh, A. Roy (eds.), *Clinical Rounds in Hepatology*,
https://doi.org/10.1007/978-981-16-8448-7_7

51

Q. What is the syndromic diagnosis of this case?

In a patient with significant alcohol intake, the presence of jaundice followed by ascites within a period of 4 weeks in the presence of encephalopathy suggests the diagnosis of Acute on Chronic Liver Failure (ACLF).

Q. What was the origin of the term acute on chronic liver failure?

Although previously used sporadically in literature the dawn of the 20th century ushered in the new concept of "Acute on Chronic Liver Failure." In a seminal paper, Sen et al. in 2002 suggested a new syndrome which they attempted to define as; *"An acute deterioration of liver function over a period of two-four weeks usually associated with a precipitating event leading to severe deterioration in clinical status with jaundice and HE and /or HRS with a high SOFA and APACHE II scores"*[3] (Sen S, et al. 2002).

Q. What are the different nomenclature systems in ACLF?

There are multiple systems and definitions that have been used to define ACLF. The following are the key definitions as defined by different societies:

1. The **Asian Pacific Association for the Study of the Liver (APASL)** originally defined ACLF in 2009 as an "**acute hepatic insult**, manifesting as **jaundice** (serum bilirubin $\geq$5 mg/dL) **and coagulopathy** (INR $\geq$1.5 or prothrombin activity <40%), complicated within **4 weeks by ascites and/or encephalopathy** with previously diagnosed or undiagnosed liver disease."

   In 2014, the definition has been modified to include the term "associated with a high 28-day mortality.

2. The second group that has proposed a definition for ACLF is the **European Association for the Study of the Liver (EASL)—Chronic Liver Failure (CLIF) consortium.** The presence of underlying cirrhosis is an essential prerequisite of this diagnosis and the scoring system is essentially centered around organ failures which are defined as:
   - Liver failure: Total bilirubin >12.0 mg/dL.
   - Kidney failure: Serum creatinine >2.0 mg/dL or the requirement of renal replacement therapy.
   - Cerebral failure: West-Haven HE Grade 3 or 4.
   - Coagulation failure: INR >2.5 or platelets are <20 × 10^9/L.
   - Circulatory failure: Vasopressor requirement (dopamine, dobutamine, epinephrine, norepinephrine, terlipressin).
   - Respiratory failure: PaO/FiO$_2$ ratio is <200 or the SpO$_2$/FiO$_2$ ratio is <214.

   Based on the organ failures, ACLF is classified into the following grades:

- **ACLF-1:**
  - Single organ kidney failure.
  - Single failure of the liver, coagulation, circulation, or respiration with serum creatinine 1.5–1.9 mg/dL (kidney dysfunction) and/or mild to moderate hepatic encephalopathy.
  - Single cerebral failure with kidney dysfunction.
- **ACLF-2 occurs in patients with 2 organ failures.**
- **ACLF-3 occurs in patients with 3 or more organ failures.**

The other factors that are incorporated in calculating the CLIF-C-ACLF and are important in determining prognosis are **age and white blood cell count at presentation.**

3. The third group that has defined and classified ACLF is the **North American Consortium for the Study of End-stage Liver Disease (NACSELD) consortium,** which proposed a definition of ACLF based upon two **or more organ failures** which are defined as:
   - Kidney: Requirement of dialysis.
   - Brain: West Haven grade 3 or 4 HE.
   - Respiratory: Requirement of mechanical ventilation or BiPAP.
   - Circulatory: Need for pressor support, MAP <60 mm Hg, or a reduction in systolic blood pressure by 40 mm Hg from baseline despite adequate fluid resuscitation.

   The NACSELD differentiates between infected and noninfected cases of ACLF.
4. In view of the variations in definitions there was an attempt to unify the concept and in this context the **World Gastroenterology Organization (WGO)** has also proposed a classification system that divides ACLF into three types:
   - Type A: (non-cirrhotic) Patients with chronic liver disease that experience a sudden flare of baseline disease (for example, autoimmune hepatitis flare) or any type of liver diseases with a hepatotropic viral superinfection.
   - Type B: (compensated cirrhosis) Seen in patients with compensated cirrhosis who experience rapid decompensation after an acute insult (Alcoholic Hepatitis on the background of alcohol-related compensated cirrhosis).
   - Type C: (decompensated cirrhosis) ACLF patients with previously decompensated cirrhosis who have a new or worsening decompensation.

Q. What are the differences between the APASL Group and the EASL CLIF Consortium definitions of ACLF?
The major differences between the two key definitions of ACLF are shown in Table 7.1.

Table 7.1 Differentiating two major definitions of Acute on Chronic Liver Failure

	APASL-ACLF	EASL CLIF consortium
Definition	**Acute hepatic** insult manifesting as **jaundice and coagulopathy,** complicated **within 4 weeks** by **ascites and/or encephalopathy** in a patient with **previously diagnosed or undiagnosed chronic liver disease associated with a high 4-week mortality**	**Acute deterioration** of **pre-existing chronic liver disease** is usually related to a **precipitating event** and associated with increased mortality at 4 weeks due to **multisystem organ failure**
Duration between insult and liver failure	4 weeks	Not defined
Acute insult	Only hepatic insults	Both hepatic and extrahepatic insults
How to define chronic liver disease?	Any chronic liver disease with or without cirrhosis (excludes previously decompensated cirrhosis)	Only cirrhosis including those with past decompensated disease
Sepsis	Is a complication of liver failure	A primary precipitant of liver failure
Variceal bleed as a precipitating event	No consensus	Yes

Bonus Points

Briefly summarize the findings of the landmark EASL-CLIF acute-on-chronic liver failure in cirrhosis (CANONIC) study (Moreau R et al. gastroenterology. 2013).

- Multicentric study involving 8 European countries.
- 1343 hospitalized patients with cirrhosis and acute decompensation.
- Used the organ failure and mortality data to define ACLF grades, assess mortality, and identify differences between ACLF and AD.
- 303 had ACLF at inception (28-day mortality 33.9%) 112 developed ACLF (28-day mortality 29.7%), and 928 did not have ACLF (28-day mortality 1.9%).
- ACLF-1 had a 28-day mortality rate of 22%, ACLF-2 (2 OFs) of 32%, and ACLF-3 (3–6 OFs) of 73%.
- ACLF patients were younger, more alcoholic, had more bacterial infections, higher leukocytes and higher CRP.
- Higher CLIF-SOFA scores and leukocyte counts were independent predictors of mortality.
- Patients without a prior history of AD had unexpectedly higher numbers of organ failures, leukocyte count, and mortality.

Q. What is acute decompensation of cirrhosis and how is it different from ACLF?

Acute decompensation (AD) of cirrhosis is defined as an acute onset of large ascites, encephalopathy, gastrointestinal hemorrhage, or bacterial infection (alone or in combination) in the absence of any other significant feature. The 28- and 90-day mortality rates in patients with AD have been found to be 5% and 14%, respectively. The differences between acute decompensation and ACLF are shown in Table 7.2:

   (c.f: The two-year mortality of patients as per the natural history of cirrhosis for variceal bleeding alone (without other decompensating events), any first nonbleeding, decompensating, and or any second decompensating event are 20%, 24%, and 50–78%, respectively.)

Q. What are the proposed subtypes of Acutely Decompensated Cirrhosis?

According to a recent study, AD has been proposed to be divided into three different phenotypes:

- **Pre-ACLF:** Tend to evolve into ACLF within 90 days and have high systemic inflammation and mortality.
- **Unstable decompensated cirrhosis:** Complications of severe portal hypertension and have frequent hospitalizations which are not due to ACLF.
- **Stable decompensated cirrhosis.**

(Trebicka J et al. J Hep. 2020).

Q. What are the commonly used scoring systems that are used to stratify prognosis in patients with ACLF?

- Patients satisfying APASL definition of ACLF: AARC score.
- Patients satisfying EASL-CLIF CANONIC definition: CLIF-C-OF and CLIF-C-ACLF score.
- NACSELD score.

Table 7.2 Differentiation between ACLF and Acute Decompensation of cirrhosis

Parameter	Acute on chronic liver failure (APASL)	Acute Decompensation of cirrhosis
Presentation	Always index	Can be index or subsequent
Type of insult	Hepatic	Hepatic or extrahepatic
Interval between insult and presentation	Within 4 weeks	Up to 12 weeks
Underlying cirrhosis	May or may not be present	Always present
28-day mortality	High	Low
Systemic inflammation	High	Moderate
Prior decompensation	No	With or without decompensation

- MELD score.
- APACHE score.
- SOFC (Simple organ failure count).

Q. What Is the pathophysiological concept of ACLF different from Decompensated Cirrhosis?
The pathophysiology of this acute syndrome, which is characterized by a state of exaggerated immune response, a state of immune dysregulation, and finally a state of immune dysfunction. A representation of this understanding is shown in Fig. 7.1.

Q. What are the general measures in the management of patients with ACLF?
Nutrition: A target of 1.5–2.0 g protein/kg per day and 35–40 kcal/kg per day with a carbohydrate-predominant late evening snack.

Intensive care. Patients with ACLF need close monitoring and attention to evolution into SIRS, and subsequent hypotension and shock. Close monitoring of hemodynamics, close attention to sensorium, and volume status for the cornerstone for management. Organ failures set in fast and progress fast. So each case of ACLF needs to be considered critically ill.

Albumin: Recent data suggest pleiotropic benefits of albumin besides its standard indications of spontaneous bacterial peritonitis, AKI, and HRS. However, albumin itself comes with its baggage of causing volume overloaded state and circulatory dysfunction and again needs a closely monitored system.

Etiology specific therapies: This includes specific cases as in HBV related ACLF, autoimmune hepatitis, and corticosteroids in alcoholic hepatitis in specific cases.

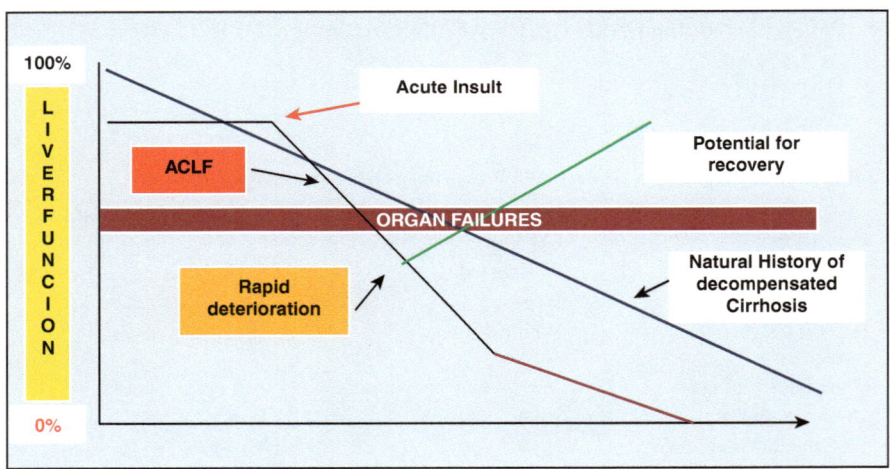

Fig. 7.1 Pathophysiological concept of ACLF

Liver transplantation (LT): The ultimate cornerstone of management in patients with ACLF remains liver transplant. This mandates an early referral to facilities with hepatology services and LT. LT in ACLF is in itself a subject of vast controversies and depends on the concept of "window to transplant" beyond which LT is possibly a futile effort.

Q. What is the role of Plasmapheresis in ACLF?
A brief overview of selected studies on plasmapheresis on ACLF is shown in Table 7.3.

Q. What are the other emerging therapies in ACLF?
Multiple strategies are being tried in ACLF and trials are underway to optimize the correct therapeutic choice.

Extracorporeal Liver support systems: Results from two multicentric studies with two different systems namely the HELIOS trial (using the Prometheus system) and the RELIEF trial (using the MARS system) did not show any benefit with regard to short-term transplant-free survival.

Fecal Microbiota Transplantation: Trials of FMT in ACLF are underway and initial results show an improvement in short-term mortality.

GCSF: GCSF has been used in settings of HBV-ACLF and as well as an overall setting of ACLF and has been shown to improve short-term survival.

Table 7.3 Overview of studies of plasmapheresis in ACLF

Authors	Etiology of cirrhosis	Duration	Volume	Results
Meng et al. 2016	HBV ACLF $n = 158$	Twice weekly 2–8 weeks	NA	• Significant decrease in bilirubin. • 28 days mortality 63% vs 82% • 3 months TFS: 18% vs 14%.
Mao et al. 2010	HBV ACLF $n = 62$	2–3 times × 2 weeks then weekly	40–60 ml/kg of plasma and 20–40 gm of albumin	30-day survival significantly better with PE (42 vs 25.2%)
Chen et al. 2015	HBV ACLF $n = 250$	Every 2–4 days	2500–3000 ml with rate of 20–25 ml/min	28-day survival Early stage ACLF:80.2% Middle stage 75.8% Late stage: 38%
Maiwal et al. 2021	65% alcohol cirrhosis $n = 131$			PE associated with Higher resolution of SIRS Lower development of multiorgan failure Lower liver failure related deaths

Bonus points: GCSF in ACLF
GCSF in HVB ACLF: Duan XZ et al. WJG. 2013
- 45 patients of HBV ACLF
- Randomized into two arms of GCSF + SOC vs standard of care (SOC).
- Dose of G-CSF: 5 µg/kg per day × 6 doses.
- Results:
Improvement in MELD/CTP scores
Improvement in 90-day survival

GCSF in ACLF: Garg V et al. Gastroenterology. 2012
- 47 patients of ACLF were randomized into two groups
- 12 doses of GCSF
- Results: In GCSF arm.
- Significant reductions in CTP/MELD/SOFA.
- Less number of patients with HE, HRS, or sepsis.
- Survival twice of that in SOC arm at 60 days.

Further Reading

Jalan R, et al. Acute-on chronic liver failure. J Hep. 2012;57(6):1336–48.
Sarin SK, et al. Acute-on-chronic liver failure: consensus recommendations of the Asian Pacific association for the study of the liver (APASL): an update. Hepatol Int. 2019;13(4):353–90.
Moreau R, et al. Acute-on-chronic liver failure is a distinct syndrome that develops in patients with acute decompensation of cirrhosis. Gastroenterology. 2013;144(7):1426–37. 1437.e1-9
Hernaez R, et al. Acute-on-chronic liver failure: an update. Gut. 2017;66(3):541–53.

Ascites and Spontaneous Bacterial Peritonitis

8

Aswath Venkitaraman, Akash Roy, and Virendra Singh

Case Vignette

A 45-year-old male presents with complaints of progressive abdominal distention and diffuse abdominal pain. He is a known case of decompensated alcohol-related cirrhosis with past decompensations in the form of ascites (diuretic responsive) and a single episode of precipitated hepatic encephalopathy. There was no history of fever, vomiting, or decrease in urine output. He has had no recent hospitalizations or medical/surgical interventions in the recent past. His physical examination is remarkable for grade II ascites.

Laboratory investigations revealed the following:

Parameter	Values	Parameter	Values
Hemoglobin	9.1	INR	1.3
Platelet count	110	HBsAg	NR
Total leukocyte count	14000	Anti HCV	Neg
Total bilirubin (Direct)	3(2.1)	Procalcitonin	1.8
AST	56	S Na/K	132/4.3
ALT	48	Albumin	3.0
ALP	91	Urea/Creatinine	44/1

Ascitic fluid analysis
Total count: 500 cells N: 80% L 20%
Protein: 1.8/Sugar 72
SAAG: 1.4

Q. What is uncomplicated ascites, and how is ascites graded?

An uncomplicated ascites is an ascites that is not associated with any of the three following features:

A. Venkitaraman · A. Roy · V. Singh (✉)
Department of Hepatology, Post Graduate Institute of Medical Education and Research, Chandigarh, Punjab, India

- Infected ascites
- Refractory ascites
- Ascites associated with the development of hepatorenal syndrome (HRS)

Ascites can be graded as follows:

Grade 1 (mild): Ascites is detected only on ultrasonography

Grade 2 (moderate): Ascites that leads to moderate symmetrical abdominal distension

Grade 3 (large or gross): Ascites that leads to marked abdominal distension

Q. What is SAAG, and how is it useful in classifying Ascites?

The acronym SAAG stands for serum-ascites albumin gradient, which helps in the subclassification of ascites into high SAAG and low SAAG ascites, respectively. SAAG is calculated by measuring the difference between albumin concentration of serum and ascitic fluid obtained on the same day. The value of SAAG of ≥ 1.1 provides an accuracy of 97% of the ascites being due to portal hypertension. The major causes of ascites classified on the basis of SAAG are shown in Table 8.1.

Q. What are the recommendations about diagnostic paracentesis in a case of New-Onset Ascites? What is the preferred site for paracentesis?

Diagnostic paracentesis is recommended in any patient with new-onset grade 2 or grade 3 ascites. An assessment of ascitic fluid cell count, total protein, and albumin concentration of the fluid as well as cultures should always be looked at once a diagnostic paracentesis is done. Assessment of additional parameters like cytology, amylase, brain natriuretic peptide levels, and adenosine deaminase should be done based on the clinical probability.

The commonest site for ascitic tap is approximately 15 cm lateral to the umbilicus with care being taken to avoid injury to liver and spleen. The inferior and superior epigastric arteries run just lateral to the umbilicus toward the mid-inguinal point and should be avoided. The preferred site is the left lower quadrant on account of a thinner abdominal wall and a comparatively greater fluid pocket. The right lower quadrant is generally avoided keeping in mind the risks of perforating a distended caecum, especially in those on laxatives.

Table 8.1 Major causes of ascites classified based on SAAG

Causes of high SAAG (≥ 1.1) ascites	Causes of low SAAG (< 1.1) ascites
Portal hypertension	Malignant ascites
Heart failure	Tubercular ascites
Hepatic vein outflow tract obstruction	Pancreatic ascites
Hypothyroidism	Nephrotic syndrome

Q. What are the principles of management of uncomplicated Ascites?

- Grade I (mild ascites): There is limited data on its evolution, and no evidence-based recommendations have been made on its management.
- Grade II ascites: A moderate restriction of sodium intake (80–120 mmol/day, corresponding to 4.6–6.9 g of salt) is recommended. In clinical practice, this equals no added salt diet with avoidance of pre-prepared meals. Patients should be appropriately educated regarding optimizing nutrition while prescribing a low salt diet.
- In addition to dietary sodium restriction, patients with moderate ascites should be started with an anti-mineralocorticoid drug (spironolactone/potassium canrenoate) with a starting dose of 100 mg/day and increased sequentially every 72 h (100 mg additions) to a maximum dose of 400 mg/day if there is no response to lower doses.
- In patients with non-response to anti-mineralocorticoids (decrease in body weight <2 kg/week) or those developing hyperkalemia, an addition of a loop diuretic (furosemide) should be done starting at 40 mg/day to a maximum of 160 mg/day (40 mg increments).
- In a select group of patients like those with persistent or gross ascites, and where a brisk diuresis is required, an upfront use combination therapy with spironolactone and furosemide can be used.
- In those who are intolerant to spironolactone (e.g., painful gynecomastia with spironolactone) amiloride can be used as an alternative, although it has a lower response rate.
- Torsemide can be used in patients showing a weak response to furosemide.
- Targets of weight loss on diuretics: 0.5 kg/day in patients without edema and 1 kg/day in patients with edema.
- Once ascites has largely resolved, the dose of diuretics should be reduced to the lowest effective dose.
- Diuretics should be stopped in cases of severe hyponatremia (serum Na <125 mmol/L), acute kidney injury (stage IA or greater), incident hepatic encephalopathy, or incapacitating muscle cramps develop.
- Furosemide should be stopped if serum potassium levels are less than <3 mmol/L and anti-mineralocorticoids should be stopped if serum potassium levels are >6 mmol/L.

Q. What is the mechanism of sodium balance in Ascites?
The concept of sodium balance is based on the equivalence of sodium intake and loss.

If a person is restricted to an 88 mmol/day intake of sodium and is not excreting any sodium in the urine at all (hypothetical situation), the net gain of sodium per day is

- **Na (intake) – Na (loss) = Na gain/day.**
- **88 mmol/day–10 mmol (insensible loss)–0 mmol (assuming no urinary excretion) = 78 mmol/day.**
- **Fluid (weight gain)/day = Na gain/Ascitic fluid Na concentration.**
- **Now assuming ascitic fluid Na concentration = Serum sodium (at optimal conditions) = 135 mmol.**
- **Per day fluid or weight gain = 78/135=0.58.**
- **Therefore, fluid or weight gain per week = 0.58 × 7 = 4,04 liters.**
- **Thus, in case a large volume paracentesis is done (6-8 liters of fluid) it should take at least 14 days to re-accumulate the 8 liters of fluid.**
- **It should be borne in mind that these calculations are based on hypothetical prerequisites of nil urinary sodium excretion and serum sodium of 135.**

Q. How is urinary sodium excretion used to monitor treatment response in Ascites?

One of the primary targets of using diuretic therapy in patients with ascites is to ensure that adequate natriuresis occurs, which is a patient on a salt-restricted diet (88 mmol of sodium/day) amounts to a urinary sodium excretion of greater than 78 mmol/day.

Alternatively, a random spot urine sodium: potassium ratio between 1.8 and 2.5 has a sensitivity of 87.5%, specificity of 56–87.5%, and accuracy of 70–85% in predicting a 24-h urinary sodium excretion of 78 mmol/day.

Q. What are the indications for doing a Large Volume Paracentesis?

The removal of ≥5 liters of ascitic fluid in a single setting constitutes large-volume paracentesis.

LVP is the first-line therapy in patients with large ascites (grade 3 ascites), which should be completely removed in a single session.

Other indications of LVP are (Sandhu BS et al. 2005; 9:715–732):

- To relieve respiratory embarrassment due to tense ascites.
- To relieve pain abdomen due to tense abdomen or increased intra-abdominal pressure or compartment syndrome.
- Serial LVPs in refractory ascites.
- To prevent impending rupture of umbilical hernia.

Q. What is Paracentesis Induced Circulatory Dysfunction?

Paracentesis induced circulatory dysfunction (PICD), previously labelled as post-paracentesis circulatory dysfunction, is a vasomotor phenomenon seen in patients who undergo paracentesis. It is defined as:

- Increase in Plasma renin activity to more than 50% from the pretreatment level to a level greater than 4 ng/ml/h on the sixth day after paracentesis.

- **Mechanisms:**
  - Aggravated arteriolar vasodilation.
  - Acute reduction of a high intra-abdominal pressure after paracentesis promotes the accentuation of arteriolar vasodilation and results in PICD.

PICD manifests as renal failure, hyponatremia, hepatic encephalopathy, and a decrease in overall survival.

Q. What are the methods of preventing PICD? The standard method in the prevention of PICD is an infusion of albumin administered at a dose of 6–8 gm/liter of fluid removed during large-volume paracentesis. In patients who are undergoing paracentesis with volume <5 L post-paracentesis, albumin infusion may not be necessary (AASLD guidelines; Runyon BA et al. Hepatology. 2013).

Q. What is the evolving role of the use of Albumin infusions in the Long-term Management of Ascites?
Long-term albumin infusions have been proposed to improve survival in patients with cirrhosis and ascites, especially those awaiting a liver transplant. Few recent studies have shown contradictory results with regard to the long-term use of albumin in patients with ascites (Fig. 8.1).

ANSWER Trial: Long-term albumin administration in decompensated cirrhosis: an open-label randomized trial (Carcareni et al. Lancet 2018).
- **Multicenter RCT;** $n = 440$
- **Cohort: Persistent uncomplicated ascites with first-line diuretics.**
- **Albumin dose: 40 g twice weekly for 2 weeks followed by 40 g weekly**
- **Albumin + Standard of care group:**
  - Significantly higher 18-month survival (77% *vs* 66%; $p = 0.028$)
  - 38% reduction in mortality
  - Reduced incidence of paracentesis, RA, SBP, infections, HRS 1, and HE 3–4
  - Improved quality of life
  - Fewer hospital admissions

MACHT Trial. (Sola et al. J Hepatol 2018) Midodrine and albumin for patients with cirrhosis awaiting liver transplantation.
A multicenter, randomized, double-blind, placebo-controlled trial 196 pts.
Midodrine (15–30 mg/day) and albumin (40 g/15 days) or placebo for 1 year.
Key results:
↓PRA (plasma renin activity) and aldosterone compared to placebo (renin 4.3 vs. 0.1 ng/ml.h, p <0.001; aldosterone 38 vs. 6 ng/dl, $p = 0.02$, at week 48 vs. baseline.
No significant differences between both groups in the probability of developing complications of cirrhosis during follow-up ($p = 0.402$) or one-year mortality ($p = 0.527$).

Q. How do we define and classify Refractory Ascites (RA)? RA is defined as ascites that cannot be mobilized or the early recurrence of which (i.e., after therapeutic paracentesis) cannot be satisfactorily prevented by medical therapy.

   Diuretic-resistant ascites because of a lack of response to dietary sodium restriction and adequate diuretic treatment.

Parameters	ANSWER Trial	MACHT Trial
Patients	431 (218 HA / 213 SMT)	173 (87 HA / 86 SMT)
Design	Randomized open-label	Randomized placebo-controlled
Baseline MELD score	12/13	17/18
Median duration of albumin administration	14.5months	63 days
Dosage and timing of Albumin administration	40 g twice a week for 2 weeks then 40 g once a week	40 g every 15 days (no loading dose)
Effect on serum albumin concentration	Steady and significant increase in albumin arm (0.6-0.8 g/dl)	No changes in both groups

Fig. 8.1 Comparing recent trials on long-term albumin administration in cirrhosis with ascites (Adapted from Zaccherini et al Acta Gastro-Enterologica Belgica 2019)

Diuretic-intractable ascites: because of the development of diuretic-induced complications that preclude the use of an effective diuretic dosage.

Q. What are the defining criteria for RA?
- **Treatment duration**: Intensive diuretic therapy (spironolactone 400 mg/day and furosemide 160 mg/day) for 1 week on salt restricted diet of <90 mmol/day.
- **Lack of response:** Mean weight loss of <0.8 kg over 4 days and urinary sodium output less than the sodium intake.
- **Early ascites recurrence**: Reappearance of grade 2 or 3 ascites within 4 weeks of initial mobilization.
- **Diuretic-induced complications**:

Hepatic encephalopathy: Development of encephalopathy in the absence of any other precipitating factors.

Renal impairment: Increase of serum creatinine by >100% to a value >2 mg/dl (177 lmol/L).

Hyponatremia: Decrease of serum sodium by >10 mmol/L to serum sodium of <125 mmol/L.

Hypo/hyperkalemia: Change in serum potassium to <3 mmol/L or >6 mmol/L despite appropriate measures.

Incapacitating muscle cramp

Q. Summarize the studies on the role of TIPSS in Refractory Ascites

Multiple RCTs have been done to evaluate the role of TIPSS in the management of refractory ascites. A brief summary of important studies is provided in Table 8.2.

Q. How is the diagnosis of SBP made and what are the subtypes of SBP?

The diagnosis of SBP is based on neutrophil count in ascitic fluid of >250/mm^3 (highest sensitivity). However, studies have shown that the highest specificity is with neutrophil count of >500/mm^3. Although the traditional teaching suggested that culture positivity is also a pre-requisite of making a diagnosis, recent guidelines do not require culture positivity as an essential prerequisite.

Culture Negative SBP (previously termed as CNNA culture-negative neutrocytic ascites): Neutrophil count in ascitic fluid of >250/mm^3 with negative cultures.

Bacterascites

Monomicrobial non-neutrocytic bacterascites: Ascitic fluid PMN count is <250, but the ascites fluid culture is positive for one bacterial organism.

Polymicrobial non-neutrocytic bacterascites: Ascitic fluid PMN count is <250, but the ascites fluid culture is positive for multiple organisms. This commonly occurs in the setting of traumatic gut perforation while doing paracentesis.

Q. What is the pathophysiology of SBP and what are the risk factors?

The key events in the pathophysiology of SBP center around altered intestinal permeability in cirrhosis along with concomitant small intestinal bacterial overgrowth.

Table 8.2 Summary of important studies of TIPSS in refractory ascites

Authors	Study population	Key results
Lebrec et al. 1996	RA defined by non-response to maximal diuretic therapy for × 5 days during hospitalization or ≥2 episodes of tense ascites requiring hospitalization in last 4 months	2-year overall survival: 29% in TIPSS group versus 56% in LVP group Increased rates of HE in uncovered TIPSS group
Rossle et al. 2000	55% of patients with RA as per IAC criteria 45% with recurrent ascites	Improved control of ascites in TIPSS group Nonsignificant improvement in 2-year transplant-free survival in TIPSS group No differences in HE rates
Gines et al. 2002	$N = 119$ Cirrhosis with RA as per IAC criteria	1-year transplant-free survival 41% against 26% in SOC arm More incidence of severe HE with uncovered TIPSS
Sanyal et al. 2003	$N = 109$ Cirrhosis with RA as per IAC criteria	Better transplant-free survival and lower recurrence of ascites in TIPSS group
Bureau et al. 2017	$N = 62$ Recurrent tense ascites defined as two LVPs in prior 3 weeks	Use of covered TIPSS leads to no differences in incident HE 1-year transplant-free survival 93% with uncovered TIPSS

In this setting, there is translocation of gut bacteria to the regional mesenteric lymph nodes. These bacteria can translocate into the systemic circulation and then reach the ascitic fluid or the mesenteric lymph nodes may rupture in the setting of increased portal pressures.

- Advanced liver disease represents one of the key risk factors for SBP.
- Previous history of SBP is associated with the risk of recurrent SBP.
- In patients who have not experienced a previous episode the following parameters have been shown to predict the risk of SBP (hence candidates of primary prophylaxis):
  - CTP score ≥ 9
  - Bilirubin ≥ 3 mg/dl
  - Creatinine ≥ 1.2 mg/DL, Blood urea nitrogen ≥ 25 mg/dL
  - S. sodium ≤ 130 mEq/l
  - Ascitic fluid total protein of < 1.5 g/dL

Ascitic fluid in SBP: Fact snippet

- Studies have shown that paracentesis for SBP is done in only 61% cases of whom it is recommended.
- Patients who received a paracentesis have 24% reduction in-hospital mortality.
- Patients with SBP with delayed paracentesis (>12 h) after admission have a 2.7-fold higher mortality.
- Direct bedside inoculation of AF sample into blood culture bottles is recommended.
- Simultaneous AF and blood culture is also recommended.
- One PMN should be subtracted from the total count for every 250 red blood cells per mm^3.
- SAAG of >1.1 g/dL predicts portal hypertensive ascites in 97% of cases and in cases SAAG of <1.1 g/dL SBP is unlikely.
- **Runyons criteria for secondary peritonitis:** Neutrocytic ascites with at least two of three criteria: ascitic fluid total protein >1 g/dL, glucose <50 mg/dL, or LDH >225 mU/mL.

Q. What is Difficult to Treat SBP?

Although not a universally accepted terminology any patient with a nosocomial SBP which is resistant to recommended empirical treatment as per local practices as well as patients with SBP having risk factors for higher mortality (severe liver dysfunction and renal dysfunction at diagnosis of SBP) are considered to have difficult to treat SBP.

Further Readings

European Association for the Study of the Liver. EASL Clinical Practice Guidelines for the management of patients with decompensated cirrhosis. J hep. 2018;69(2):406–60.

Moore KP, et al. The management of ascites in cirrhosis: report on the consensus conference of the International Ascites Club. Hepatology. 2003;38(1):258–66.

Aithal GP, et al. Guidelines on the management of ascites in cirrhosis. Gut. 2021;70:9–29.

Arka De, Akash Roy, and Virendra Singh

Case Vignette

A 40-year-old male presents with complaints of progressive abdominal distention associated with pain and a decrease in urine output. He is a known case of decompensated alcohol-related cirrhosis with past decompensations in the form of ascites (diuretic responsive) and a single episode of precipitated hepatic encephalopathy. There is a history of fever for the last two days, which is concomitant with abdominal pain. There is no history of vomiting, facial puffiness, swelling of legs, or cardiorespiratory embarrassment. He has had no recent hospitalizations or medical/surgical interventions in the recent past. His physical examination is remarkable for grade III ascites. In the hospital, he has a BP of 100/60 mm Hg and pulse rate of 100/min, and a urine output of 300 ml over the last 24 h.

Laboratory investigations revealed the following:

Parameter	Values	Parameter	Values
Hemoglobin	8.1	INR	1.5
Platelet count	120	HBsAg	NR
Total leukocyte count	13000	Anti-HCV	Neg
Total bilirubin (Direct)	4(3.1)	Procalcitonin	3
AST	56	S Na/K	127/4.3
ALT	48	Albumin	2.9
ALP	91	Urea/Cr	60/2.1

Ascitic fluid analysis
Total count: 500 cells N: 80% L 20%
Protein: 1.8/Sugar 72
SAAG: 1.4

A. De · A. Roy · V. Singh (✉)
Department of Hepatology, Post Graduate Institute of Medical Education and Research, Chandigarh, Punjab, India

© The Author(s), under exclusive license to Springer Nature Singapore Pte Ltd. 2022
V. Singh, A. Roy (eds.), *Clinical Rounds in Hepatology*,
https://doi.org/10.1007/978-981-16-8448-7_9

Q. What is the overall syndromic diagnosis?

Given the background of the patient, this is a case of Decompensated Alcohol-Related Cirrhosis with complications in the form of Spontaneous Bacterial Peritonitis, Acute Kidney Injury, and Hyponatremia.

Q. What was the traditional definition of AKI in cirrhosis?

Traditionally, AKI in cirrhosis has been centered around serum creatinine (S.cr) and was conceptually framed into two primary contexts:

- In patients without baseline renal impairment: Increase in serum creatinine level by more than 50% of the baseline value **and e**xceeding 1.5 mg/dl.
- In patients with pre-existing renal impairment: Increase in serum creatinine by more than 50% above the baseline value.

Q. What is the Acute Kidney Injury Network (AKIN) criteria for AKI?

According to the Acute Kidney Injury Network (AKIN), AKI is defined as an abrupt (≤48 h) reduction in kidney function manifested by either:

- Rise in serum creatinine level of more than 0.3 mg/dl (26.5 µmol/l) in 48 h.
- Rise in serum creatinine≥50% (by a factor of 1.5 from baseline).
- Decrease in documented urinary output (UO)(<0.5 ml/kg body weight/h for >6 h).

In the KDIGO modification, all parameters are the same as AKIN with the addition of a 7-day period for a 50% rise in Cr.

Q. How is AKI staged?

AKI stage	Serum Cr criteria	Urine output (UO) criteria
I	Increase of S.Cr by ≥0.3 mg/dl or increase to 1.5–1.9 times from baseline	UO <0.5 ml/kg/h for 6–12 h
II	Increase of S.Cr to 2.0–2.9 times from baseline	UO <0.5 ml/kg/h for ≥12 h
III	• Increase of S.cr ≥3.0 times from baseline or • S.Cr ≥4.0 mg/dl or RRT or • In patients <18 years, decrease in estimated GFR to <35 ml/min per 1.73 m²	UO <0.3 ml/kg/h for ≥24 h or anuria for ≥12 h

Q. What are the potential causes of AKI in cirrhosis?

Pre-renal	Intrinsic renal	Post renal
Volume depletion Gastrointestinal (G.I). bleed, G.I. loss, diuretic, sepsis	**Acute tubular necrosis (ATN)** Ischemia, sepsis, toxins, drugs, radiological contrast	**Obstructive nephropathy**
Decreased effective perfusion HRS Cardiorenal syndrome NSAIDs, Cox-2 inhibitors, radiological contrast	**Glomerular disease**	
	Interstitial disease	

- Although this is a general classification, it should be understood that there may be a rapid transition from pre-renal to ischemic ATN in patients with shock.
- Also, in certain selected cases with impaired renal autoregulation mechanisms and afferent arteriolar pathologies like endarteritis/arteriosclerosis, there may be a state of ischemic ATN with only a borderline decrease in arterial pressure.

Q. What is the importance of urine analysis in the diagnosis of AKI in cirrhosis?

One of the key steps in the approach to AKI in cirrhosis is to perform a thorough urine analysis. The key indicators that should be looked into while performing urine analysis are shown in Table 9.1.

Q. What are the points of differentiation between Pre-renal and Intrinsic Renal Disease (ATN)?

Principle: The capacity of the renal tubules to reabsorb sodium and to concentrate urine is preserved in pre-renal AKI and impaired in ATN. Although there are possibilities of overlap between the two entities the fundamental points of difference between the two entities is shown in Table 9.2.

Q. What is the classical definition of hepatorenal syndrome (HRS), and what are its modifications?

Originally, the concept of HRS was proposed as **Sassari's Criteria of HRS in 1978.** Although the basic principles of diagnosis have remained the same, the definitions have undergone modifications. The International Club of Ascites defines HRS has proposed several definitions which evolved to the **2015 definition which defines HRS as a type of AKI defined as:**

- Diagnosis of cirrhosis and ascites
- Diagnosis of AKI according to International Club of Ascites (ICA-AKI) criteria
- Non-response to 2 consecutive days of diuretic withdrawal and volume expansion with albumin 1 g/kg bodyweight
- Absence of shock

Table 9.1 Key findings in urine analysis

Indicators	Possible pathologies
Pigmented granular casts	Toxic or Ischemic ATN
Red cell casts	Glomerulonephritis
Significant proteinuria	Glomerulonephritis

Table 9.2 Key points in differentiating types of AKI

Parameter	Pre-renal AKI including HRS-1	ATN
Urine microscopy	No casts Urine sediments±	Granular/epithelial casts
Urine osmolality	>500 mOsm/kg	<350 mOsm/kg
Urine sodium	<10 mEq/l	>20 mEq/l

- No concurrent nephrotoxic drugs
- No macroscopic evidence of structural kidney injury is defined as:
  - No proteinuria (>500 mg/day)
  - No microhematuria (>50 red blood cells per high power field)
  - Normal renal ultrasonography

However, it is important to note that the HRS-AKI criteria came with a corollary that even who satisfy the criteria of HRS-AKI may still have an element of tubular damage, and in such cases, urine biomarkers have a role to more accurately differentiate HRS from acute tubular necrosis.

Q. What Is the old classification of HRS-1 and HRS-2, and what are the current concepts in defining and classifying HRS AKI?
According to older concepts and definitions, HRS was traditionally classified as:

Type I HRS
At least a twofold increase in serum Cr to a level greater than 2.5 mg/dL over a period of <2 weeks without sustained improvement in renal function (<20% decrease in Cr) at least 48 h after diuretic withdrawal and albumin challenge.

Type II HRS
A slowly progressive form of renal impairment is seen in the setting of advanced cirrhosis and refractory ascites characterized by avid sodium retention.

However, with the advent of the newer definitions of the International Club of Ascites, these classifications have now been considered obsolete.

According to the newer concept and consensus, HRS which satisfies the ICA definition of HRS can have the subtypes in cirrhosis as shown in Table 9.3.

Q. What are the potential biomarkers to differentiate HRS from ATN?
Multiple biomarkers have been studied, of which the most significant ones include:

Urinary neutrophil gelatinase-associated lipocalin (u-NGAL): Cut-off for best predictive accuracy for distinguishing ATN-AKI from HRS-AKI is 220 ug/g Cr. Approximately 88% of the patients with HRS-AKI have values below this cut-off.

Table 9.3 Newer definition in the diagnosis of HRS

HRS AKI (Previously HRS-1)	• ΔIncrease in S.Cr $\geq$0.3 mg/dl within 48 h and/or • UO$\leq$0.5 ml/kg B.W. $\geq$6 h or • Increase in S.Cr $\geq$50% from baseline (lowest available in last 3 months)
HRS NAKI (not AKI) Previously HRS-2	
HRS AKD	• eGFR <60 ml/min per 1.73 m^2 for <3 months in the absence of structural causes • Increase in SCr <50% from baseline (lowest available in last 3 months)
HRS-CKD	• eGFR <60 ml/min per 1.73 m^2 for $\geq$3 months in the absence of structural causes

Fractional excretion of Urinary Sodium (FeNa): Conventionally, in nephrology practice, FeNa has been long used to distinguish between pre-renal AKI and ATN. However, in cirrhosis, on account of avid sodium retention, even patients with ATN tend to have a FeNa <1%, thus making the differentiation difficult. However, recent literature suggests that lower cut-offs (<0.2%) of FeNA may be useful for differentiating ATN-AKI from HRS-AKI.

Other potential biomarkers include:

- Cystatin C
- Interleukin-18 (IL-18)
- Kidney Injury Molecule-1 (KIM-1)
- Liver-type fatty acid-binding protein (L-FABP)

Q. What is the role of vasoconstrictor therapy in HRS?

Vasodilation with resultant decreased effective arterial blood volume (EABV) is the cornerstone of HRS pathophysiology. Therefore, the principle of therapy is the replenishment of intravascular blood volume with albumin as well as the use of vasoconstrictors. The principle vasoconstrictors used are shown in Table 9.4.

Q. Provide a Brief Comparison of the Effectiveness of Vasoconstrictors in HRS

Table 9.5 summarizes the major studies of the effectiveness of different vasoconstrictors in HRS.

Table 9.4 Characteristics of vasopressors used in HRS

Vasoconstrictor	Mechanism of action	Dosage
Terlipressin	• Vasopressin analog • V1 receptors on vascular smooth muscles • Exert maximum effect on mesenteric and cutaneous circulation	0.5 mg IV 4–6 hourly If no response can increase to 1 mg/4–6 hourly
Noradrenaline	• Alpha plus beta-adrenergic agonist • Vasoconstriction in the peripheral circulation (limited effect on splanchnic circulation) and an increase in cardiac output	0.5–3 mg/hr as infusion Target is an increase in MAP by ≥ 10 mm/Hg
Octreotide + Midodrine	**Octreotide:** • Inhibits release of glucagon as well as other vasodilatory molecules • It also has a direct vasoconstrictive effect on splanchnic and the systemic circulation • Vasoconstriction of portosystemic collaterals	50 mcg bolus followed by 50 mcg/hr continuous IV infusion
	Midodrine: Alpha-1 agonist leads to systemic as well as splanchnic vasoconstriction	7.5 mg three times daily can be increased up to 15 mg thrice daily Targets MAP≥ 10 mmHg or MAP>80 mmHg

Table 9.5 Major studies of vasoconstrictor effectiveness in HRS

Study	Intervention arm	Control arm	30 day-mortality	Reversal of HRS
Terlipressin vs. Placebo/Control				
Solanki et al. 2003	Terlipressin 1 mg/12 h × 15 d (+albumin); $N = 12$	Placebo × 15 d (+albumin); $N = 12$	Terlipressin: 7/12 Placebo: 12/12	Not reported
Sanyal et al. 2008	Terlipressin 1 mg/6 h up to 2 mg/6 h × 14 d (+albumin) $N = 56$	Placebo × 14 d (+albumin); $N = 56$	Terlipressin: 32/56 Placebo: 35/56	Terlipressin: 19/56 Placebo: 7/56
Noradrenaline (NA) vs Terlipressin				
Sharma et al. 2008	NA 0.5 mg/h up to 3 mg/h × 15 d (+albumin) $N = 20$	Terlipressin 0.5 mg/6 h up to 2 mg/6 h × 15 d (+albumin) $N = 20$	NA: 9/20 Terlipressin: 9/20	NA: 10/20 Terlipressin: 8/20
Singh et al. 2012	NA 0.5 mg/h up to 3 mg/h until HRS reversal or a maximum of 14 d (+albumin) $N = 23$	Terlipressin 0.5 mg/6 h up to 2 mg/6 h until HRS reversal or a maximum of 14 d (+albumin); $N = 23$	NA: 15/23 Terlipressin: 16/23	NA: 10/23 Terlipressin: 9/23
Octreotide + Midodrine vs. Terlipressin				
Cavallin et al. 2015	Midodrine.7.5 mg/8 h up to 12.5 mg/8 h + Octreotide s.c. 100 μg/8 h up to 200 μg/8 h until HRS reversal or a maximum of 14 d (+albumin) $N = 22$	Terlipressin 3 mg/24 h up to 12 mg/24 h until HRS reversal or a maximum of 14 d (+albumin) $N = 27$	Octreotide +Midodrine: 7/22 Terlipressin: 8/27	Octreotide+Midodrine: 1/22 Terlipressin: 15/27
Octreotide + Midodrine vs. Noradrenaline (NA)				
Tavakkoli et al. 2012	Midodrine 5 mg × 3/day up to 15 mg × 3/day + octreotide 100 μg/8 h up to 200 μg/ 8 h until HRS reversal or a maximum of 15 d (+albumin); $N = 9$	NA 0.1 μg/Kg/min up to 0.7 μg/Kg/min until HRS reversal or a maximum of 15 d (+albumin); $N = 6$	Octreotide + Midodrine: 4/9 NA: 4/6	Octreotide + Midodrine: 6/9 NA: 5/6

Q. What is the role of terlipressin infusion in the management of HRS?

In a study by Cavallin et al., it was shown that Terlipressin given as infusion had a few advantages over bolus terlipressin, which include:

- Lower rate of adverse events (35.39% vs. 62.16%; $p<0.025$)
- Similar treatment response (76.47% vs 64.85%)
- Lower mean daily dose (2.23 6 0.65 versus 3.51 6 1.77 mg/day; $P<0.05$) (Table 9.6)

Q. What are the potential predictors of response to terlipressin therapy?

Baseline Cr <5 mg/dl
>   Baseline bilirubin <10 mg/dl
>   Early increase in MAP (5 mm Hg at day 3)

Q. What are the results of the CONFIRM trial?

Despite extensive use in European and Asian populations, Terlipressin has not been granted US-FDA approval. The CONFIRM trial was a recent large-scale randomized controlled trial for the use of Terlipressin in HRS-AKI with 300 patients in northern America.

Key features:

- Sick patients (average MELD 33).
- Baseline serum Cr: 3.5 mg/dl in both groups.
- Dose of Terlipressin: 1 mg every 6 hourly for 14 days.
- The primary endpoint as verified HRS reversal (VHRSR): 2 consecutive Cr values of ≤ 1.5 mg/dL at least 2 h apart.
- VHRSR was seen in 29.1% in the terlipressin group compared to 15.8% in the placebo ($p=0.01$).
- 90-day survival without transplant was similar (~28% in each group).

Q. If there is non-response to vasoconstrictor therapy, what are the next management options?

There are two approaches toward the next step management of HRS, which are non-responsive to standard vasoconstrictor therapy.

Table 9.6 Use of Terlipressin as infusion vs. bolus in HRS

	Infusion regimen	Bolus regimen
Initial dose	2 mg/24 h	0.5 mg q 4 hourly
Escalation of dose	Serum Cr decrease < 25% at 48 h	
Maximum dose	12 mg/24 h	2 mg q 4 hourly
Definitions of response		
– Partial	>50% decrease in serum Cr but final value >1.5 mg/dl	
– Complete	Cr<1.5 mg/dl	
Maximum duration of therapy	24 h after attainment of complete response or 15 days	

Novel combination therapies: Sequential noradrenaline in addition to Terlipressin.

Non-medical management:

Transjugular intrahepatic portosystemic shunt (TIPSS) has been shown to have a role in reversing HRS in selected studies. Results from a pooled meta-analysis suggest a short-term survival of 72%, which reduces to 47% at 1 year. These studies report a high rate of hepatic encephalopathy (49%), which has raised concerns regarding the use of TIPSS in this situation.

Renal Replacement therapy: The use of RRT in patients with HRS who are already on vasoconstrictor plus albumin therapy has been studied in limited studies. One retrospective study of 80 patients found no difference in 30- or 180-day survival. At this stage, RRT may only be used as a bridge to liver transplantation.

Further Readings

European Association for the Study of the Liver. EASL clinical practice guidelines on the management of ascites, spontaneous bacterial peritonitis, and hepatorenal syndrome in cirrhosis. J Hep. 2010;53(3):397–417.

Angeli P, et al. Diagnosis and management of acute kidney injury in patients with cirrhosis: revised consensus recommendations of the International Club of Ascites. Gut. 2015;64(4):531–7.

Angeli P, et al. News in pathophysiology, definition and classification of hepatorenal syndrome: a step beyond the International Club of Ascites (ICA) consensus document. J Hep. 2019;71(4):811–22.

Hepatic Encephalopathy

10

10

Rohit Mehtani, Akash Roy, and Virendra Singh

Case Vignette A 52-year male presents with alcohol-related cirrhosis with previous history of variceal gastrointestinal bleed and ascites now presents with irrelevant talk and disorientation. The family had noticed a behavioral change with slowing of mentation and not sleeping at night of late and has been constipated. He has been off alcohol for the last 6 months and medications include diuretics, non-selective beta-blockers, lactulose, and zinc supplementation. He has a BMI of 19.2 kg/m². He is afebrile and has a BP 9/60, PR 110/min, and RR 22/min. His physical exam is remarkable for multiple spider angiomas and presence of asterixis. There is no focal neurological deficit. Per abdominal examination is remarkable only for the presence of free fluid. A non-contrast CT brain was ordered in the emergency which reveals. His blood investigations are as shown in the below table.

Laboratory investigations revealed the following:

Parameter	Values	Parameter	Values
Hemoglobin	9.2	INR	1.5
Platelet count	77	HbSAg	NR
Total leukocyte count	9000	Anti-HCV	Neg
Total bilirubin (Direct)	2.1(1.2)	S Na/K	121/4.3
AST	62	Urea	56
ALT	34	Creatinine	1.2
ALP	91	Albumin	3.1

R. Mehtani · A. Roy · V. Singh (✉)
Department of Hepatology, Post Graduate Institute of Medical Education and Research, Chandigarh, Punjab, India

© The Author(s), under exclusive license to Springer Nature Singapore Pte Ltd. 2022
V. Singh, A. Roy (eds.), *Clinical Rounds in Hepatology*, https://doi.org/10.1007/978-981-16-8448-7_10

Q. What is the probable diagnosis and how do you classify it?

The probable diagnosis on the basis of history is Type C Overt (Grade II) Episodic Precipitated (constipation) Hepatic Encephalopathy in a patient with decompensated alcohol-related cirrhosis. Hepatic encephalopathy is classified as per different axes which include:

Axis 1: Etiology

Type A: In **A**cute liver failure

Type B: In cases with predominant portosystemic shunting (**B**ypass physiology)

Type C: In patients with **C**irrhosis

Axis II: Clinical Severity

Unimpaired

Covert HE: Comprises both minimal HE + West Haven Grade I (absence of disorientation and asterixis).

Overt HE: Comprises West Haven Grades II–IV HE

Axis III: Time Course

Episodic: Episodes ≥6 months apart

Recurrent: 2 episodes within 6 months

Persistent: Presence of behavioral alterations that are persistently present with intermittent relapses of overt HE.

Axis IV: Precipitated or Spontaneous

Spontaneous

Precipitated (secondary to)

Q. What are the key clinical pointers towards suspecting a diagnosis of Hepatic Encephalopathy? What are the mimics of HE?

The key indicators toward suspecting a diagnosis of HE lies in clinical suspicion in a patient with suspected liver disease, absence of alternative causes and adequate response to therapy.

An algorithmic approach is provided below:

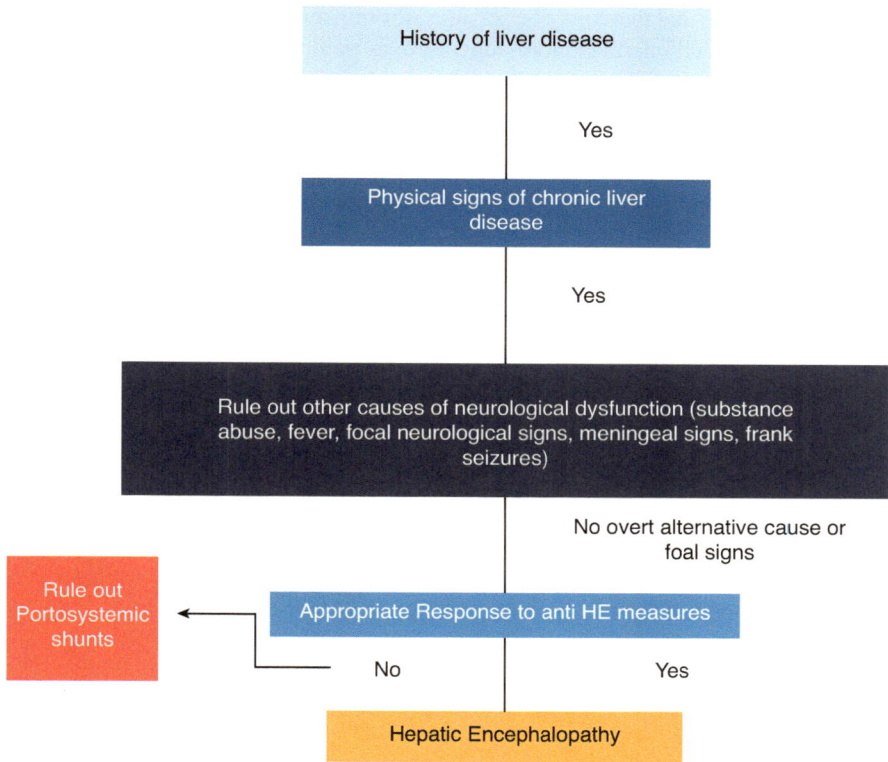

The common clinical presentations which may mimic HE and should be ruled out are:

- Dyselectrolytemia (note hyponatremia can be concurrent with HE)
- Alcohol intoxication, Wernicke's encephalopathy, alcohol withdrawal, delirium tremens
- Encephalitis
- Sepsis-associated encephalopathy
- Cerebrovascular accidents
- Myxedema coma

Q. How do you distinguish between HE and alcohol withdrawal?
The validated score for alcohol withdrawal that needs therapeutic intervention is the *Clinical Institute Withdrawal Assessment of Alcohol Scale, Revised (CIWA-Ar) score.* However, the score has specifically not been validated in alcoholic cirrhosis and may be influenced even in presence of mild grades of HE. The timing of withdrawal is variable and although most commonly seen after 48–72 h of alcohol cessation it may occur up to a week after last alcohol intake. Tremulousness is usually

a cardinal feature and there may be seizures. Prominent restlessness, agitation, auditory, visual, or tactile hallucination may serve as pointers. However, clinical differentiation is at times difficult from hepatic encephalopathy.

Q. What are the tests for assessment of Minimal Hepatic Encephalopathy (MHE)?

PHES: The International Society for Hepatic Encephalopathy (ISHEN) recommends the Psychometric Hepatic Encephalopathy Score (PHES) score diagnosis of MHE. The test comprises 5 paper pencil tests that measure psychomotor processing speed and visual-motor coordination.

- Number Connection Test A (NCT A)
- Number Connection Test B (NCT B)
- Digit Symbol Test (DST)
- Line Tracing Test (LTT)
- Serial Dotting Test (SDT)

Animal naming test (ANT): It is a simple bedside test with enumeration of a maximum number of animals in a time span of 1 minute. A score of less than 10 is considered abnormal. The ANT is influenced by extremes of age and educational status.

Continuous reaction time (CRT): This is a computerized test where the auditory stimulus is given through a headphone and the time to response (button press) is recorded. The normal value is provided by the CRT index which if below 1.9 may be suggestive of MHE.

The inhibitory control test (ICT): This is a computerized test that involves identifying specific letters (X, Y) in sequence and to avoid responding to any other sequence. In the ICT a "lures" is defined as a repetitive same sequence like (X followed by an X instead of Y).

Critical flicker frequency (CFF): This is a psychophysical test and is based on the concept of retinal gliopathy as an indicator of HE. The principle is based on the frequency at which a flickering light (from 60 Hz downward) is observed. The advantage of this test is its ability to quantify HE as well as objectivity.

Stroop Test: This is a neuropsychological test available in the form of an application "Encephalapp" which is based on Stroop Effect originally described by John Ridley Stroop in 1935. The test is based on the concept of a mismatch between the name of a color (e.g., "blue," "green," or "red") and the color in which it is depicted ("red" shown in blue color instead of red color itself).

Q. What is the West Haven classification and what are the stages in it?

The West Haven classification is a classification system developed for grading stages of HE originally formulated by Professor Harold Conn and colleagues while evaluating the therapeutic efficacy of lactulose. It has the following grades:

- **Grade 0**: No obvious changes but has potentially underlying mild decrease in intellectual ability and coordination (Minimal Hepatic encephalopathy).
- **Grade 1:**
  - Minor lack of awareness
  - Euphoria or anxiety
  - Shortened attention span
  - Impaired performance of calculations
  - Altered sleep rhythm
- **Grade 2:**
  - Lethargy or apathy
  - Minimal disorientation for time or place
  - Subtle personality change
  - Inappropriate behavior
  - Dyspraxia and presence of asterixis
- **Grade 3:**
  - Somnolence progressing to stupor, but responsive to verbal stimuli
  - Confusion
  - Gross disorientation
  - Bizarre behavior
- **Grade 4:** Coma

Q. What is the role of ammonia level measurement in clinical practice?

Although, ammonia is one of the central drivers of the pathophysiology of HE its role in diagnostic and prognostic significance has been controversial.

Principles of ammonia testing

- Arterial or venous blood are comparable
- Venous blood should be drawn in fasting state, kept on ice packs, and examined within 30–60 mins.
- If capillary method is used earlobe is the best site as sweat may interfere with fingerpick capillary sample results.
- Whichever method is used appropriate calibration and reference normal values should be standardized.

The role of ammonia in the diagnosis of HE in cirrhosis is not as clearly established as in acute liver failure. For staging patients with HE, ammonia levels tend to be higher with higher stages of HE but there remains a considerable overlap between the stages and there are no absolute cut-off values. For prognosis, hyperammonemia has been associated with increased rates of hospitalizations, breakthrough episodes, and mortality.

Factors affecting ammonia levels

- High-protein diet intake
- Prolonged fasting due to muscle breakdown or intense physical activity
- Gastrointestinal bleeding

- Presence of renal dysfunction
- Post TIPSS

Q. What are the treatment strategies for patients with HE?

The current guidelines focus on the type of presentation of encephalopathy and broadly define treatment strategies as follows:

Covert HE: Once covert HE is diagnosed there is an increased risk for the development of overt HE. Hence, current guidelines recommend lactulose therapy in patients who test positive for CHE on an individualized basis. Pooled meta-analysis data also shows that lactulose is the only beneficial agent for both prevention of progression of MHE as well as its reversal (Dhiman RK Clin Gastroenterol Hepatol. 2019 S1542- 3565(19)30969-3).

Acute episode of overt HE

Carefully look for precipitants of HE and correct them

1st choice: Lactulose either by enema or oral route based on patient profile.

Intravenous L-Ornithine L-Aspartate can be used as an alternative or additional agent to treat patients nonresponsive to lactulose.

Polyethylene glycol can also be used in case of ileus or prior intolerance to lactulose.

Prevention of recurrence

Lactulose is recommended for the prevention of recurrence of OHE.

Rifaximin is recommended as an add-on to lactulose for prevention of recurrent OHE.

Q. What is the evidence for other additional therapies in the management of HE?

Multiple agents have been used as additional therapy in the management of HE which include:

Probiotics: Have been shown to improve recovery as well as delay time to second hospitalization in patients with HE but has no proven benefit on mortality.

Branched-chain amino acids: BCAA have been shown to have some beneficial effects in the prevention of recurrent HE as well as an additional agent in refractory HE.

Zinc: Zinc is an important cofactor in several key enzymatic cycles and zinc deficiency is common in cirrhosis. However, zinc supplementation has only been shown to improve psychometric tests.

L-ornithine-L-aspartate: Available in both intravenous and oral forms and can be used as an add-on therapy in patients not responding to conventional therapy.

A schematic representation of pharmacotherapeutic usage in HE is shown in Fig. 10.1.

Q. Describe in brief the Emerging Therapies in HE

Polyethylene glycol (PEG): PEG has been shown to be efficacious in the improvement of HE in patients who were already on lactulose (Shehata HH Eur J Gastroenterol Hepatol 2018; 30:1476–81).

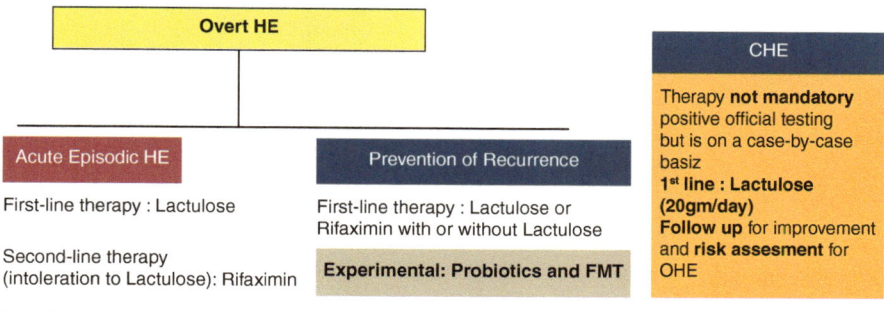

Fig. 10.1 Schematic representation of pharmacotherapy for Hepatic Encephalopathy

Intravenous albumin: Intravenous albumin in combination with lactulose has been shown to be more effective than lactulose alone for the complete reversal of HE (Sharma BC et al . J Gastroenterol Hepatol 2017).

Ornithine phenylacetate and glycerol phenylbutyrate act as ammonia scavengers and have been shown to lower ammonia levels.

Fecal microbiota transplantation (FMT): FMT has been shown to prevent the recurrence of HE in a small randomized trial.

Further Reading

Häussinger D, Schliess F. Pathogenetic mechanisms of hepatic encephalopathy. Gut. 2008 Aug 1;57(8):1156.

Ortiz M, Jacas C, Córdoba J. Minimal hepatic encephalopathy: diagnosis, clinical significance and recommendations. J Hepatol. 2005 Apr 1;42(1):S45–53.

Vilstrup H, Amodio P, Bajaj J, Cordoba J, Ferenci P, Mullen KD, Weissenborn K, Wong P. Hepatic encephalopathy in chronic liver disease: 2014 Practice Guideline by the American Association for the Study of Liver Diseases and the European Association for the Study of the Liver. Hepatology. 2014 Aug;60(2):715–35.

Bajaj JS, Lauridsen M, Tapper EB, Duarte-Rojo A, Rahimi RS, Tandon P, Shawcross DL, Thabut D, Dhiman RK, Romero-Gomez M, Sharma BC. Important unresolved questions in the management of hepatic encephalopathy: An ISHEN consensus. Am J Gastroenterol. 2020 Jul 1;115(7):989–1002.

Approach to Variceal Hemorrhage

Arun Valsan, Akash Roy, and Virendra Singh

Case Vignette

A 40-year-old male, an alcohol consumer (120 gm/day for 5 years) now presents episode of hematemesis followed by alteration in sensorium. There are no other significant medical comorbidities. There is no history suggestive of abdominal distention, decreased urine output, shortness of breath. On examination he is hypotensive (BP 90/55 mmHg), has tachycardia (HR 126/min) deeply icteric, and has parotid enlargement with bilateral pedal edema. There is presence of asterixis. Per abdominal examination is remarkable for an enlarged firm irregular liver.

Laboratory investigations revealed the following:

Parameter	Values	Parameter	Values
Hemoglobin	10.2	INR	2.1
Platelet count	120	HbSAg	NR
Total leukocyte count	14000	Anti-HCV	Neg
Total bilirubin (Direct)	6 (4.2)	S Na/K	129/4.3
AST/ALT	144/62	Urea	74
ALP	91	Creatinine	1.3
Albumin	3.2	S Na/K	129/4.3

USG abdomen: Liver (16 cm) with coarse echotexture and an enlarged spleen. The gallbladder and biliary system were unremarkable. Portal vein diameter was 13 mm. Spleen 12 cm. There is no free fluid.

Q. What is meant by clinically significant Portal Hypertension (CSPH)?

CSPH represents an advanced stage of portal hypertension which is defined as an hepatic venous pressure gradient (HVPG) >10 mmHg. CSPH is central to the development and progression of varices. In patients with compensated cirrhosis without

A. Valsan · A. Roy · V. Singh (✉)
Department of Hepatology, Post Graduate Institute of Medical Education and Research, Chandigarh, Punjab, India

83

varices, varices develop at the rate of 5–8% depending upon the degree of CSPH. In these patients with CSPH careful distinction should be made between those with no/small varices and those with high-risk varices.

Q. What are the risk factors for poor outcomes during an episode of Acute Variceal Bleed (AVB)?
When a patient presents with an episode of AVB certain indicators are there which tend to predict the prognosis of the patient. These include

HVPG: Those with HVPG >20 mmHg have 5 times increased risk of failure to control bleed or have early rebleeding leading to higher 6-week mortality.

Child-Pugh Score: The CTP score and Child class although a broader prognostic indicator also add to the stratification of patients with AVB. Approximately 80% of Child C patients have an HVPG >20 mmHg, which in turn is associated with poor outcomes following AVH. On the contrary, patients belonging to Child class A have excellent outcomes.

Therapy for portal hypertension: Once AVH has occurred rebleeding risks are higher in those not receiving portal pressure reducing agents (60% vs 30%). Similarly lowering HVPG to lower than 12 mm Hg leads to a very low risk of rebleed.

Associated decompensating event: The presence of ascites and or HE increases the overall mortality in patients with AVB. D'Amico et al have shown that when VH is the only decompensating event mortality is 20%, whereas when it is associated with ascites or encephalopathy mortality increases to 88% (D'Amico et al Alimentary Pharmacotherapeutics' 2014).

Q. Classify Portal Hypertension as Per Hepatic Venous Pressure Gradient
The HVPG values are key in differentiating types of portal hypertension and a simplistic way of approaching the same is shown in Table 11.1.

Q. What are the options for primary prophylaxis for preventing initial Variceal Hemorrhage?
Prophylaxis is indicated for medium/large varices irrespective of CTP class or for small high-risk varices with red wale signs or for small varices with CTP C stage. The two modalities that are available as per recommendations for primary prophylaxis are nonselective beta-blockers or endoscopic variceal ligation till variceal

Table 11.1 Portal hypertension on the basis of HVPG values

Axis	WHVP	FHVP	HVPG (WHVP-FHVP)
Prehepatic	N	N	N
Presinusoidal	N	N	N
Sinusoidal	Increased	N	Increased
Post sinusoidal	Increased	N	Increased
Post Hepatic	Increased	Increased	±

WHVP Wedged hepatic venous pressure, *FHVP* Free hepatic venous pressure, *HVPG* Hepatic venous pressure gradient

eradication. Traditional NSBB (propranolol, nadolol) and carvedilol are the recommended first-line options with carvedilol being more effective than traditional NSBB in HVPG reduction. As per the currently available evidence there is no clear added benefit of combination EVB and NSBB therapy and hence not recommended.

A comparison of propranolol and carvedilol is provided in Table 11.2.

Q. Provide a Schematic Outline of the Management of a Patient with AVH? (Fig. 11.1)

Table 11.2 Comparison between properties of beta-blockers in the management of portal hypertension

Propranolol	Carvedilol:
Mechanism of action: β1 (decrease cardiac output) and in β2 (reduction splanchnic blood flow) blockade	**Mechanism of action:** β1 (decrease cardiac output) and in β2 (reduction splanchnic blood flow) block with additional α-1-blockade and nitric oxide production (decrease intrahepatic resistance and produces intrahepatic and systemic vasodilatation)
Dosage: 20–40 mg orally twice a day	
Maximal dosage: 320 mg/day	**Dosage:** To initiate with 6.25 mg once a day
Side effects:	**Maximal dosage:** 12.5 mg/day
Bradycardia	**Side effects:**
Fatigue	Fatigue
Bronchoconstriction	Initial exacerbation of heart failure
Cardiac failure	Renal dysfunction
Dizziness	
Impotence (?)	

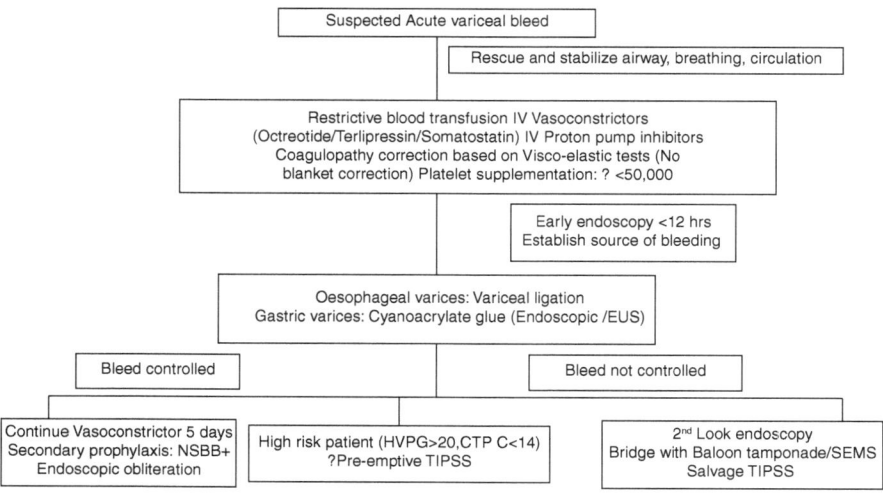

Fig. 11.1 Simplified approach to a patient with Acute Variceal Bleed

Q. Describe in brief the study advocating restrictive transfusion strategies in Acute GI Bleed

The comparison between restrictive versus liberal transfusion strategies in acute GI bleed was shown in a randomized control trial in which a subgroup of 921 patients with cirrhosis, 461 were randomized to the "restrictive-strategy" (transfusion at threshold of 7 g/dL with target range after transfusion of 7–9 g/dL) and 460 to the "liberal-strategy" transfusion at threshold of transfusion of 9 g/dL with a target of 9–11 g/dL). In the analysis, it was seen that the probability of survival was significantly higher with restrictive transfusion strategy in patients with Child class A or B but not in those with Child class C (HR = 1.04, 95% CI = 0.45–2.37). Additionally, patients in the liberal-strategy group had a significant increase of HVPG (from 20.5 ± 3 to 21.4 ± 4 mmHg, $p = 0.003$) despite the administration of somatostatin (Villanueva C et al. N Engl J Med. 2013).

Q. What is the role of antibiotic prophylaxis in patients with Variceal Hemorrhage?

VH has been shown to be associated with an increased risk of infection which in turn leads to an increased risk of hemostasis failure and mortality. Antibiotic prophylaxis has been shown to reduce mortality, incident infections, early rebleeding, and overall hospital stay.

Antibiotic of choice: Depending upon patient profile and local antimicrobial profile.

Fernandez et al in an RCT comparing ceftriaxone with norfloxacin had shown that the probability of developing overall infections or SBP, or spontaneous bacterial peritonitis was significantly higher in patients receiving norfloxacin. In this context, Ceftriaxone (1 g/24 h) is the first choice in patients with the following parameters: (Fernández J et al Gastroenterology. 2006):

- Advanced cirrhosis: 2 or more of ascites, severe malnutrition, encephalopathy, or bilirubin >3 mg/dL.
- Patients on quinolone prophylaxis.
- Settings with a high prevalence of documented quinolone resistance.

Q. What are the options for vasoactive therapy in patients with VH?

The available drugs that have been used as vasoactive agents include:

- Terlipressin (intravenous): 1–2 mg every 4 h until control of bleeding; then 1 mg every 4 h maintenance. Caution to be exerted in view of side effects including arrhythmia, tissue ischemia, and potential development of hyponatremia.
- Somatostatin (intravenous): Initial bolus of 250 µg followed by continuous infusion of 250–500 µg/hr.
- Octreotide (intravenous): Initial bolus of 50 µg followed by continuous infusion of 50 µg/hr.

Q. Define failure to control bleeding in patients presenting with AVB

Failure in controlling AVB may occur in 10–15% of patients presenting with AVB. It is defined as death or need to change therapy due to one of the following:

- Fresh hematemesis or nasogastric aspiration of ≥100 ml of fresh blood ≥2 h after the start of a specific drug treatment or therapeutic endoscopy.
- Development of hypovolemic shock.
- 30 g/L drop in hemoglobin (9% drop of hematocrit) within any 24 h period if no transfusion is given.

Q. Describe the role of Balloon Tamponade and Stents in the management of Refractory Variceal Bleed

Sengstaken–Blakemore tube (SBT) or Linton-Nachlas balloon (LNB) are options for mechanistic balloon tamponade therapy to stop refractory bleeding. Although success can be achieved in up to 90% of the cases, the primary drawback of this therapy is chances for rebleed of up to 50% of the cases. Other associated complications like aspiration, migration of the device, and necrosis/perforation of the esophagus are not infrequent. Hence, such measures are better undertaken in an intensive care setting with adequate monitoring.

An alternate to balloon tamponade devices is Self Expanding Metal Stents (SX-ELLA Danis). In one study with patients with refractory VB use of this SEMS controlled VB in 79.4% (27/34) of patients (Pfisterer N et al Liver International. 2019). In a single RCT comparing SEMS to balloon tamponade therapy, it was found that control of bleeding was higher while transfusion requirements and adverse events were lower in SEMS group (Escorsell et al. Hepatology 2016).

Q. What is the role of rescue and pre-emptive TIPSS in management of Acute Variceal Bleed?

In spite of adequate therapy 10–15% of patients presenting with AVB may have persistent bleeding or early rebleeding which is associated with increased mortality.

Factors associated with failure of primary therapy (Abraldes JG et al. Journal of Hepatology. 2008):

- HVPG (>20 mmHg)
- CTP C
- WBC>10 × 10^9/L,
- Presence of portal vein thrombosis
- Systolic blood pressure at admission <100 mmHg

In such cases, if bleeding is persistent after a second look endoscopy then the use of TIPSS as a measure for control of bleed is called 'Rescue TIPSS"

In contrast to this "Pre-emptive TIPSS" is based on the hypothesis that an early placement of TIPSS in patients who are at high risk would lead to improvement in survival.

The criteria that have been used to classify patients at high risk are:

- $HVPG \geq 20$
- CTP B with active bleed on endoscopy
- CTP C <14

Q. Classify Gastric Varices

Gastric varices are seen in up to 20% of patients with cirrhosis with a bleeding incidence of 25% at 2 years. Bleeding events tend to be more frequent as well as of higher severity and also have a higher risk of rebleed in comparison to esophageal varices. The classification most commonly used in gastric varices is summarized below:

GOV1: Esophageal varices extending below cardia into lesser curvature (Most common).

GOV-2: Esophageal varices extending below cardia into fundus (2nd most common; Bleeding risk greater than GOV 1).

IGV-1: Isolated varices in the fundus (Maximum bleeding risk).

IGV-2: Isolated varices else in the stomach.

Q. What are the management options for management of patients with Gastric Variceal Bleed?

The principles of management of bleeding from gastric varices are the same as esophageal varices, which include maintenance of hemodynamic stability, resuscitation, and early endoscopy. Injection therapy with cyanoacrylate ("glue") is recommended as the endoscopic hemostatic treatment when GOV2 or IGV varices are considered the source of hemorrhage. The modality for glue injection can be endoscopic or endoscopic ultrasound (EUS) guided.

For prevention of rebleed from gastric varices, the options include repeated sessions of cyanoacrylate injection, nonselective beta-blockers, TIPSS, or balloon-occluded retrograde transvenous obliteration (BRTO). On comparing glue injection to NSBB for prevention of gastric variceal rebleeding in patients with GOV2 with eradicated esophageal varices or IGV1 rebleeding in the cyanoacrylate group has been seen to be significantly lower (Mishra et al Gut 2010). In a recent study, in patients with history of bleeding from GOV-2 or IGV-1 randomized to either cyanoacrylate injection or BRTO treatment it was seen that the probability of rebleeding was higher in the cyanoacrylate injection group (Luo et al Hepatology. 2021).

Q. What is the role of TIPSS in management of Gastric Variceal bleed?

TIPS has shown to be effective in the treatment of bleeding from GOV2 or IGV1. Currently, there are no head-to-head trials of TIPSS vs endoscopic glue therapy as the primary modality. Hence, the choice of endoscopic glue therapy vs. TIPSS based upon current evidence needs to be individualized depending upon availability/expertise of either modality, presentation, overall disease severity, contraindications, and associated comorbidities (EASL 2018). With respect to prevention of rebleed, one RCT comparing cyanoacrylate injection and TIPSS found rebleeding from gastric varices to be less common post TIPSS (Lo et al. Endocopy 2007).

Further Reading

de Franchis R. Evolving Consensus in Portal Hypertension Report of the Baveno IV Consensus Workshop on methodology of diagnosis and therapy in portal hypertension. J Hepatol. 2005 Jul 1;43(1):167–76.
De Franchis R. Expanding consensus in portal hypertension: Report of the Baveno VI Consensus Workshop: Stratifying risk and individualizing care for portal hypertension. J Hepatol. 2015 Sep 1;63(3):743–52.
European Association for The Study of the Liver. EASL Clinical Practice Guidelines for the management of patients with decompensated cirrhosis. J Hepatol. 2018 Aug 1;69(2):406–60.

Autoimmune Hepatitis

Akash Roy, Virendra Singh, and Ashim Das

Case Vignette

A 23-year-old female from Himachal Pradesh with medical history for thyroid disease consuming Levothyroxine (50 ucg) now presents with deranged liver functions as an outpatient consult. Past medical history is significant for two episodes of jaundice which was self-resolving in the past 1.5 years. She has no other medical or surgical history. There is no history of any drug or complementary/alternative medical history. Her family history is unremarkable. Physical exam shows a BMI of 20.2 kg/m^2 presence of sclera icterus with mild pallor. There are no peripheral stigmata of chronic liver disease. Per abdominal examination is unremarkable.

Laboratory investigations revealed the following:

Parameter	Values	Parameter	Values
Hemoglobin	9.1	INR	1.2
Platelet count	164	HBsAg	NR
Total leukocyte count	9000	Anti-HCV	Neg
Total bilirubin (Direct)	4 (3.1)	ANA/ASMA	++/+
AST	344	S Na/K	13/4.3
ALT	410	Urea/creatinine	21/0.9
ALP	100	Total Ig G	2700 mg/dl
Albumin	3.4	Ig M HAV/HEV	Negative

A. Roy · V. Singh (✉)
Department of Hepatology, Post Graduate Institute of Medical Education and Research, Chandigarh, Punjab, India

A. Das
Department of Pathology, Post Graduate Institute of Medical Education and Research, Chandigarh, Punjab, India

V. Singh, A. Roy (eds.), *Clinical Rounds in Hepatology*, https://doi.org/10.1007/978-981-16-8448-7_12

Q. What is the probable clinical diagnosis and what further test will you like to order?

In the setting of a young female, with background thyroid disorder and history of intermittent jaundice with current presentation of significantly elevated transaminases and a positive autoimmune serology the most probable diagnosis is autoimmune hepatitis (AIH). However, to establish the diagnosis a liver biopsy will be the next test.

Q. What are the diagnostic scoring systems for AIH and what are the advantages of each of these scoring systems?

The original diagnostic scoring system was proposed in 1993 by the International Autoimmune Hepatitis Group (IAIHG). This was subsequently revised in 1999 (Table 12.1). However, for diagnostic simplicity a simplified scoring system has

Table 12.1 Revised International Autoimmune Hepatitis Group (IAIHG) Scoring System

Criteria	Score	Criteria	Score
Gender If Female	+2	**HLA DRB1*03 or DRB1*04 positive**	+2
ALP: AST or ALT ratio		**Alcohol Use**	
>3	−2	<25 gm/day	+2
<1.5	+2	>60 gm/day	−2
ANA/SMA or LKM 1		**Liver biopsy**	
>1:80	+3	Interface Hepatitis	+3
1:80	+2	Plasmacytoid infiltrate	+1
>1:40	+1	Hepatic rosettes	+1
1:40	0	No specific feature	−5
AMA if positive	−4	Biliary Changes	−3
		Fat, Granuloma others	−3
Gamma globulin levels	−4	**Concurrent immune disease** (thyroiditis, colitis, etc.)	+2
>2 ULN	+3		
1.5-2 ULN	+2		
1-1.4 ULN	+1		
Viral Markers	−3	**Other liver-related markers (anti-SLA, anti actin)**	+2
Positive	+3		
Negative			
Hepatotoxic drugs		**Response to treatment**	
Yes	−4	Complete response	+2
No	+1	Relapse	+3

Pretreatment score:
Definite diagnosis **>15**
Probable diagnosis **10–15**

Posttreatment score:
Definite diagnosis **>17**
Probable diagnosis **12–17**

Table 12.2 Simplified International Scoring System for the Diagnosis of Autoimmune Hepatitis

Criteria	Interpretation	Score
ANA or SMA	>1:40	+1
Anti LKM	>1:80	+2
Anti SLA	>1:40	+2
	Positive	+2
Immunoglobulin G Levels	>ULN	+1
	>1.1ULN	+2
Histology		
Interface Hepatitis with no incompatible findings	Compatible with AIH	+1
Interface Hepatitis with lymphoplasmacytic infiltration	Typical of AIH	+2
Viral Markers (HBV, HCV, HAV)	Negative	+2
Aggregate score: Definite diagnosis ≥7 Probable diagnosis **6**		

been introduced since 2008 (Table 12.2). The applications of the two scoring systems are more complementary than exclusive. While in a classical clinical setting with typical features the simplified scoring system can be enough to clinch the diagnosis, in more complicated phenotypic presentations the detailed scoring system is required to enable a definitive diagnosis.

Revised IAIHG Scoring System **Mnemonic** **SAAG- is HER-GOD**		
S = Sex (female) **A: Alcohol** **A: Antibodies** **G: Globulins**	**H-Histology** **E-Enzymes** **R-Response to treatment**	**G-Genetics** **0-Others** **D:Drugs**

Q. What are the limitations in the diagnostic scoring systems for AIH?

• Lack of validation in specific groups like acute severe AIH and AIH presenting as ALF.
• Unproven accuracy in the setting of overlap syndrome, concomitant NAFLD or post-liver transplant AIH.
• Reliance on immune-fluorescence than ELISA for serological markers.

Q. What are the classical clinical presentations of AIH?

AIH has a wide variety of presentations ranging from asymptomatic chronic hepatitis to decompensated cirrhosis to presentations like fulminant hepatic failure (Table 12.3). It is important to recognize these entities as each has its own natural history and therapeutic approaches with individual nuances.

Table 12.3 Common clinical presentations of AIH

Presentation	Key features
Asymptomatic	• 25–35% of patients • 25–75% become symptomatic within a mean duration of 32 months • Do not have spontaneous biochemical or histological improvement • May have histology akin to symptomatic patients
Chronic hepatitis	• Seen in one-third of the patients • Most commonly present with fatigue, malaise, arthralgias, or amenorrhea • Most common presentation is easy fatigability • Jaundice may be present in certain cases
Cirrhosis	• Seen in up to 25–30% of the patients at presentation
Acute severe AIH and AIH-ALF	• **AS-AIH**: Jaundice, INR>1.5<2, no encephalopathy in a patient without previously recognized chronic liver disease • **AIH-ALF:** Jaundice, INR>2 with hepatic encephalopathy in a patient without previously recognized chronic liver disease • Acute presentation is defined as <30 days from onset • Variably reported in 25–75% cases depending upon individual series • **ANA is absent or weakly positive in 29–39%** • **Ig G levels are normal in 25–39%** • **4 cardinal features in AIH-ALF histology are:** – Central perivenulitis (65%); – Plasma cell-enriched inflammatory infiltrate (63%); – Massive hepatic necrosis (42%) – Lymphoid follicles in (32%).

Q. What are the concurrent extrahepatic diseases associated with AIH? What are the recommendations for screening such Diseases?

• Concurrent extrahepatic autoimmune diseases are seen in around 14–44% and are seen more commonly in women, patient with HLA DRB1*04:01, and those having a positive family history.
• Most common: Autoimmune thyroid disease.
• Others include:
  – Type 1 DM.
  – Autoimmune skin disorders (vitiligo, urticaria, alopecia areata, and leukocytoclastic vasculitis).
  – Ulcerative colitis.
  – Pernicious anemia.
  – Rheumatoid arthritis.

AIH and Celiac Disease

Celiac disease is seen more commonly in patients with AIH than in general population. Frequency has been reported to be variable ranging from 2.8 to 16%. Besides AIH itself, concomitant presence of liver involvement due to celiac disease itself may lead to liver dysfunction. It is suggested that children with AIH and celiac who are in remission do better if they are also on a GFD than those still on a gluten-containing diet.

Guideline recommendations (AASLD 2019)

- All patients with AIH should be **screened** for celiac and thyroid diseases at diagnosis.
- AIH patients should be **assessed** for rheumatoid arthritis, IBD, autoimmune hemolytic anemia, diabetes, and other extrahepatic autoimmune conditions.

Q. How do you differentiate between Type 1 and Type II AIH? What is the relevance of the differentiation in clinical practice?

Based on certain clinical characteristics and autoimmune markers AIH has been subtyped in Type and Type II (previously also Type III). However, it must be borne in mind that there is considerable overlap in the phenotypes and treatment approaches and hence its clinical relevance is limited.

Characteristics	Type 1 AIH	Type II AIH
Age group	More commonly in adults	Seen more commonly in children (However, even in children overall Type I AIH>Type IIAIH)
Type of presentation	Chronic presentation is more common	Frequently tend to present with acute presentations
Cirrhosis at presentation	Adults: 28–33% Children <33%	Rarer
Frequent antibodies	ANA SMA, anti-actin SLA	Anti-LKM1
Presentations as overlap syndrome	More common especially in adults	Rarely seen
Need of long-term steroid therapy	In certain cases, remission may be achieved off steroids	Relapses are frequent thus mandates long-term immunosuppression

Bonus points: All about antibodies and AIH	
Cardinal Markers	
Type I AIH	ANA, ASMA
Type II AIH	LKM
In adults at presentation	
ANA (antinuclear antibody)	80%
ASMA (anti-smooth muscle antibody)	60%
LKM (liver-kidney-microsomal antibody)	3%
Multiple antibodies	50%
In children at presentation LKM	13–30%
Other ANA Positivity	PSC, NAFLD, CHC, CHB, Cirrhosis
Other ASMA Positivity	PSC, CHC, ALD
Anti SLA (soluble liver antigen)	Specific for Type I AIH Severe disease Predictor of relapse
anti-actin, anti-α-actinin	Acute severe AIH in Type 1 Incomplete response Relapse
Anti-liver cytosol type 1 (LC-1)	Children with severe AIH

Q. What are the histological hallmarks of classical AIH?

- Interface hepatitis is a hallmark for diagnosis of AIH and is accompanied by lobular (panacinar) hepatitis (50%) and plasma cell infiltration (two-thirds).
- Centrilobular (zone 3) necrosis may be an early or severe histological stage, coexists with interface hepatitis in 78%, and can also be seen in those with accompanying cirrhosis.
- Emperipolesis (65%).
- Hepatocyte rosettes (33%).
- IgG4-positive plasma cells may be present but its significance is poorly understood.
- Concomitant NAFLD/NASH may be seen in 20–30% of the cases.
- Prominent biliary changes (bile duct destruction, ductopenia) or atypical (e.g., granulomas, copper, or iron) should invoke the search for other etiologies.

Q. What are the common drugs that are associated with drug-induced AIH-like Injury?
Most common: Minocycline, Infliximab, Nitrofurantoin, and methylDopa (**MIND**).

Probable association: Statins (**R**osuvastatin, **A**torvastatin) **Pr**opylthiouracil, **I**soniazid **D**iclofenac [**RAPID**].

Newer agents: Immune checkpoint inhibitors (Both CTLA-4 and PD-1/PDL-1 inhibitors), Adalimumab.

Q. What are the key approaches to differentiate between AIH and Drug-induced AIH-like Injury?
The key historical and clinical indicators of differentiation are:

- DILI-AIH is always acute onset (although time from exposure to manifestation may be delayed) whereas AIH can present both as chronic hepatitis as well as an acute hepatitis picture.
- Temporal association with a potentially implicating drug is the key to DILI-AIH.
- Markers for hypersensitivity like rash, fever, eosinophilia, and urinary eosinophils are more common with DILI-AIH than AIH.
- Concomitant presence of other autoimmune disorders indicate more toward AIH.
- Both need to be treated with steroids. However, relapse after withdrawal of steroids in a suspected case almost always proves AIH.
- If biopsy is done presence of extensive high fibrosis or cirrhosis indicated more toward AIH.

Q. What is the role of transient elastography in noninvasive fibrosis assessment in AIH?
Vibration controlled transient elastography (VCTE) commercially available as Fibroscan has a good correlation with fibrosis stage in AIH. However, in the

early stages of the disease the correlation may be improper due to ongoing inflammation. Therefore, once inflammation has been adequately reduced (6 months of adequate immunosuppression) the following are the cut-offs of VCTE in AIH:

kPa 5.8: ≥F2 fibrosis
kPa 10.5: ≥F2 fibrosis
kPa 16: ≥F3 fibrosis

Q. What are the indications of treatment in patients with confirmed AIH?

AIH is a lifelong disease and therapy if initiated is often lifelong. The balance lies between the efficacies of therapy versus to prevent disease progression versus therapy-associated side effects.

All patients with evidence of **moderate or severe inflammation**, those who have **cirrhosis and active disease, symptomatic patients,** and **younger patients** (to prevent cirrhosis) are candidates for therapy.

Elderly patients with mild disease activity and/or **significant comorbidity** (decompensated **burnt-out cirrhosis**) where the **risk of immunosuppression outweighs** the benefit may not be candidates of therapy.

According to the **2010 AASLD guidelines,** the following are the **absolute recommendations** for AIH treatment:

- AST >10× ULN
- AST >5× ULN and gamma globulin >2× ULN
- Bridging or multiacinar necrosis on histology
- Incapacitating symptoms

Also, the following were considered as conditions that **do not warrant treatment:**

- Asymptomatic with normal AST and globulins
- Inactive cirrhosis, mild portal inflammation
- Severe cytopenia
- TPMT deficiency
- Pathologic fractures, psychosis, uncontrolled diabetes, or hypertension

Note: 2019 AASLD guidelines: All patients with AIH are candidates for therapy except individuals with inactive disease by clinical, laboratory, **and** histological assessment.

Q. What are the First-line recommendations for treatment in AIH?

The first-line recommended treatment is prednisolone/prednisone alone or in combination with azathioprine.

Dosage:

Prednisone: When used alone 40–60 mg daily in adults and 1–2 mg/kg daily in children (maximum dose 40–60 mg daily) or a lower dose of prednisone, 20–40 mg daily, in combination with AZA).

Azathioprine: 50–150 mg daily or 1–2 mg/kg daily; pediatric dosing: 1–2 mg/kg daily.

Example of regimen (EASL guidelines on AIH 2015) for a 60 kg adult

Duration from onset	Prednisolone	Azathioprine
1	60	–
2	50	–
3	40	50
4	30	50
5	25	100
6	20 .	100
7 + 8	15	100
8+9	12.5	100
10	10	100

• A lower dose of initial prednisolone may be used in case of mild disease.

• Reduction of prednisolone to 7.5 mg/day if aminotransferases normalize and after three months to 5 mg/day, tapering out at 3–4 months intervals depending on patient's risk factors and response.

• According to some groups AZA can be started simultaneously as glucocorticoids.

• Most, however, recommend waiting 2 weeks before starting AZA to confirm **steroid responsiveness, evaluate TPMT status**, and exclude the **rare possibility of AZA-induced hepatitis.**

Q. What is the role of checking TPMT activity while using Azathioprine? What are the other assessments to be made while patient is on corticosteroid therapy?

TPMT activity is useful in identifying some rare (0.3–0.5%) patients with zero or nearly undetectable who may develop severe myelosuppression on Azathioprine. Although not universally recommended assessment of TPMT activity may be done prior to AZA initiation.

Other considerations prior to initiation of immunosuppressive therapy include:

• Vaccination of HAV and HBV.

• Patients who are HbsAg negative but anti-HBc positive should be periodically assessed and closely monitored for HBV reactivation while on a standard steroid dose in combination with AZA.

• However, if patient is receiving high-dose steroids or B-cell depleting agents the then preemptive HBV therapy should be considered.

• Careful assessment of bone mineral density, Vitamin D status, and features of metabolic syndrome.

Bonus points: Response criteria's in AIH

Previous definitions (Muratori et al Hepatology 2009)
Complete response: Disappearance of symptoms (if present) and biochemical remission (i.e., normal transaminase and gammaglobulin levels) with very low doses of steroids (2–4 mg/day of methylprednisolone or equivalent.
Partial response: Despite a higher dose of steroids and associated azathioprine transaminases <2× ULN) without achieving complete normalization.
Nonresponse: Persistently elevated (>2 ULN) transaminase levels, despite "intensive immunosuppression."

Newer recommendations (AASLD 2019)
Biochemical Remission: Normalization of serum AST, ALT, and IgG levels (IgG levels may be elevated once cirrhosis sets in).
Histological Remission: Absence of inflammation in liver tissue after treatment.
Incomplete Response: Improvement of laboratory and histological findings that are insufficient to satisfy criteria for remission.
Relapse: Exacerbation of disease activity after induction of remission and drug withdrawal (or non-adherence).
Treatment Failure: Worsening laboratory or histological findings despite compliance with standard therapy.
Treatment Intolerance: Inability to continue maintenance therapy due to drug-related side effects.

Q. What are the alternative drugs that have been used as First-line Therapy in AIH?

Budesonide (advantage of having 90% first pass metabolism) has been used in combination with AZA has been shown to have equal efficacy as prednisolone plus AZA with the advantage of lesser side effects. It appears to have an extremely safe profile in pediatric AIH. However, as cirrhosis sets in the side effect sparing effect of budesonide may be lost and the trials involving budesonide primarily have not included acute severe AIH and patients with cirrhosis. Portal vein thrombosis is also a potential side effect of budesonide use which needs to be looked at carefully.

Q. What are the potential predictors of poor response to initial therapy in AIH?

Onset at an early age, acute presentation, hyperbilirubinemia, HLA DRB1*03, cirrhosis at diagnosis, and a high initial MELD score have been found as potential indicators of therapeutic failure. High levels of Anti-actin, elevated ferritin levels (>2.1-fold ULN) have also been proposed as indicators of nonresponse.

Q. What are the second-line therapies in AIH?

The drugs that have been used as second-line agents in patients with AIH include mycophenolate mofetil, cyclosporine, calcineurin inhibitors, 6-mercaptopurine, and biologics (rituximab and infliximab).

Further Reading

Lohse AW, Chazouilleres O, Dalekos G, Drenth J, Heneghan M, Hofer H, Lammert F, Lenzi M. EASL clinical practice guidelines: autoimmune hepatitis. J Hepatol. 2015 Oct 1;63(4):971–1004.

Volk ML, Reau N. Diagnosis and management of autoimmune hepatitis in adults and children: a patient-friendly summary of the 2019 AASLD guidelines. Clin Liver Dis. 2021 Feb;17(2):85.

Hennes EM, Zeniya M, Czaja AJ, Parés A, Dalekos GN, Krawitt EL, Bittencourt PL, Porta G, Boberg KM, Hofer H, Bianchi FB. Simplified criteria for the diagnosis of autoimmune hepatitis. Hepatology. 2008 Jul;48(1):169–76.

Manns MP, Czaja AJ, Gorham JD, Krawitt EL, Mieli-Vergani G, Vergani D, Vierling JM. Diagnosis and management of autoimmune hepatitis. Hepatology. 2010 Jun;51(6):2193–213.

Primary Biliary Cholangitis

13

Saurabh Mishra, Akash Roy, and Virendra Singh

Case Vignette

A 45-year-old female presented with a history of new onset of generalized weakness, fatigue, and pruritis for past 6 months. There was no history of any prodrome, fever, abdominal pain, prior biliary surgery, or recent complementary medication intake. There is no history of alcohol consumption, substance abuse, tattooing, or high-risk sexual behavior. On physical examination, she had scleral icterus and skin excoriations due to itching. Per abdominal examination was remarkable for an enlarged (3 cm below right costal margin) firm liver with splenomegaly.

Laboratory investigations revealed the following

Parameter	Values	Parameter	Values
Hemoglobin	9.1	INR	1.2
Platelet count	140×10^3	HBsAg	NR
Total leukocyte count	9000	Anti-HCV	Neg
Total bilirubin (Direct)	3 (2.1)	ANA/AMA	Negative/Positive
AST	92	S Na/K	134/4.3
ALT	56	Urea/creatinine	21/0.9
ALP	446	p-ANCA	Negative
Albumin	3.4	Ig M HAV/HEV	Negative
USG abdomen	Liver enlarged 16 cm mildly irregular in outline with increase echogenicity. Spleen 11 cm. No ascites small GB calculi		

S. Mishra · A. Roy · V. Singh (✉)
Department of Hepatology, Post Graduate Institute of Medical Education and Research, Chandigarh, Punjab, India

© The Author(s), under exclusive license to Springer Nature Singapore Pte Ltd. 2022
V. Singh, A. Roy (eds.), *Clinical Rounds in Hepatology*, https://doi.org/10.1007/978-981-16-8448-7_13

Q. What is the most probable diagnosis?

The clinical presentation is suggestive of a cholestatic liver disorder and given the age and AMA seropositivity the most probable diagnosis is primary biliary cholangitis.

Q. Explain in brief the approach to Cholestatic Disorders of the Liver?

Cholestasis results from an impairment of bile formation and/or bile flow and has a wide spectrum of presentation including fatigue, pruritus, and jaundice. Traditionally, cholestasis is subdivided into **two broad categories, intrahepatic cholestasis (IC) and extrahepatic cholestasis (EC)**. While in IC the abnormalities are predominantly at the hepatocellular level or at the level of small bile ducts obstructive lesions in the medium to large bile ducts lead to EC.

Patients with cholestasis can **present in two ways**, i.e., **asymptomatic or symptomatic**. Asymptomatic cases are detected on the basis of abnormalities in LFTs while symptomatic patients may present with features such as fatigue, pruritus, and jaundice.

The first step toward a biochemical diagnosis of cholestasis is an elevated alkaline phosphatase (>1.5 ULN). As ALP can have multiple sources of production, in cases of diagnostic uncertainty, addition of gamma-glutamyl transpeptidase levels (>3 ULN) supports the diagnosis of cholestasis.

The second step in the evaluation of cholestasis is the differentiation between IC and EC. Detailed clinical history and physical findings serve as important indicators toward differentiation. Features like history of cholangitis (biliary pain, fever), vomiting, history of prior biliary surgery, features of gastric outlet obstruction are pointers toward an extrahepatic cause. A detailed history of alcohol, drug, and herbal supplements intake, recurrent fluctuating cholestasis, family history of cholestasis should be obtained.

The third step involves imaging with Ultrasonography (US) as the initial test of choice to differentiate intra-from extrahepatic cholestasis.

Additional work-up is dependent on individual case findings and involves further imaging in the form of MRCP, EUS, autoantibody profile (ANA, AMA), liver biopsy, and in selected cases ERCP.

Q. How is the diagnosis of PBC Made?

Definition: Primary biliary cholangitis (PBC) previously known as Primary Biliary Cirrhosis is a rare autoimmune cholestatic liver disease that has certain cardinal features, which include **cholestasis**, serologic reactivity to **antimitochondrial antibodies (AMA)** or **specific antinuclear antibody (ANA)**, with additional histology suggestive of non-**suppurative**, **granuloma**, and **lymphocytic small bile duct cholangitis**.

PBC is diagnosed based on the history, physical findings, laboratory tests, and histology, if available.

The combination of cholestatic biochemical tests in the absence of any other cause and presence of AMA, especially in a middle-aged female is sufficient to make a diagnosis of PBC.

Q. Describe the natural history of PBC
Natural History of PBC

The natural history of untreated PBC follows a protracted course with a sequence of phases with differential rates of progression.

Preclinical or silent phase: AMA positive but biochemically silent.
Asymptomatic phase (Biochemical abnormalities only but no symptoms).

- Most of the new patients are diagnosed in this stage.
- Although this phase may be prolonged up to 20 years, on average 30–50% of patients remain asymptomatic after 5 years.

Symptomatic phase

- Most commonly present with fatigue, pruritis, hyperpigmentation, jaundice, and right abdominal pain with evidence of enlarged liver on physical exam.
- Portal hypertensive features develop subsequently.
- 20% develop ascites and 10% develop bleeding varices in a period of 10 years.

Liver failure phase
Onset of progressive jaundice heralds a pre-terminal phase.
Mean survival once the bilirubin is 2.0 mg/dl and 6.0 mg/dl is 4 years and 2 years, respectively.

Q. What are the epidemiological characteristics of PBC?
Epidemiology

- PBC is primarily a disease of **middle-aged women**.
- Peak incidence occurs in the **5th decade**, and is rare in less than 25 years of age.
- The youngest reported age of confirmed disease onset is 15 years.
- However, there has been a **trend toward earlier diagnosis** as more patients are being detected early in their natural history as asymptomatic cases during routine evaluation.
- **Female-to-male** gender ratio is around **10:1**.
- The **annual incidence** is variable and ranges from 2.27 to 32 per million.
- **Highest prevalence** has been reported from Scandinavian countries, Spain, Canada, and the UK.

Q. Describe in brief the characteristic autoantibodies associated with PBC
AMA

- A hallmark of PBC is the presence of **anti-mitochondrial antibodies (AMAs)**, which are characteristic of PBC and are present in 90–95% of the cases.
- AMAs are a group of antibodies reacting to different mitochondrial antigens.

- AMA PDH-E2 is the major and most specific AMA directed against the E2 component of the mitochondrial ketoacid dehydrogenase complexes (Pyruvate dehydrogenase).
- Other AMA like Anti-M4, anti-M8, and anti-M9 are not clinically relevant.
- AMA can be determined by multiple methods including Indirect Immunofluorescence (IIF) and ELISA.
- IIF has low sensitivity, whereas ELISA has a higher sensitivity but low specificity.
- Appearance of AMA typically precede disease onset.
- AMA titers do not correlate with disease activity.

ANA (Anti-nuclear antibodies)

- ANAs are positive in around 30–50% of patients with PBC, especially those negative for AMA.
- ANA when positive, tends to be specific in PBC.
- The immunofluorescence pattern of ANA like multiple nuclear dot ANA (sp100) and membrane rim ANA pattern (gp210) are highly specific.

Other antibodies
Antibodies like anti-Kelch 12 and anti-hexokinase-1 are also specific to PBC.

Q. What are the clinical features and management strategies in PBC?
Clinical features and their respective management strategies
The majority of patients with PBC are asymptomatic at presentation and are diagnosed on the basis of screening tests and PBC-specific antibodies. When symptomatic the most common symptoms are fatigue and pruritis.
Fatigue

- Most common symptom and has been noted in up to 80% of the cases in some studies, although reporting variability differs depending on the mode of assessment.
- Associated with a significant negative impact on quality of life irrespective of disease stage or severity.
- Associated conditions that may promote fatigue include hypothyroidism, depression, anemia, sleep apnea, and restless leg syndrome.
- No specific treatment options but evaluation of associated conditions and development of coping strategies is recommended

Pruritis

- Reported in around 69% of patients with PBC.
- Associated with a significant negative impact on quality of life.
- Characteristically worse at bedtime and is more localized to palms and soles.
- Factors like retention of bile acids, increased opioidergic tone and autotoxin activity have been proposed in pathogenesis.

- Cholestyramine has been recommended as the first-line therapy.
- Rifampicin at a dose of 150–300 mg daily is recommended as a second-line agent.
- Other modalities: Anti-histaminics, opioid antagonists, sertraline, and plasmapheresis.
- Refractory pruritus: Liver transplantation has been suggested to be an option.

Osteoporosis

- *Risk factors*: Advancing age, lower BMI, severe cholestasis, and higher histological stage of disease (fivefold higher risks).
- *Mechanism*: Decreased bone formation; Bilirubin has been thought to interfere with adequate bone formation by inhibiting osteoblastic activity.
- *Screening*
  - DEXA is recommended at presentation and on follow-up to assess osteoporosis.
  - Assessment of FRAX (Fracture risk assessment tool) score.
- Reasonable to commence treatment femur T-score <1.5 with supplementation of calcium and vitamin D.
- Bisphosphonates although considered safe should be reserved for those with significantly elevated fracture risk and caution exercised in patients with varices.

Malabsorption

- Although uncommonly seen in modern era patients may still present with features nocturnal diarrhea, foul-smelling bulky stools, weight loss despite a preserved appetite.
- Features of vitamins A, D, E, K deficiencies.
- In patients with associated Sicca syndrome features of pancreatic insufficiency may be common.
- Supplementation is recommended on an individual basis.

Dyslipidemia

- Hyperlipidemia may be seen in up to 80% of cases.
- However, no substantial evidence to establish an elevated cardiovascular risk.
- Pharmacological therapy may be considered in patient with other metabolic risk factors, low HDL, and increased LDL.

Q. What are the physical examination and biochemical findings in PBC?
Physical examination findings

- Clinical findings are stage dependent.
- Hepatomegaly is an early feature.

- Splenomegaly as a part of the disease as well as an early indicator of portal hypertension (Some patients with PBC develop portal hypertension before the onset of cirrhosis).
- Skin abnormalities: Stigmata of pruritis, hyperpigmentation, xanthelasma, and xanthomas.
- As disease progresses signs of liver cell failure and portal hypertension set in.

Biochemical Features

- Elevation in serum alkaline phosphatase is the hallmark of PBC however biochemical tests alone do not make the diagnosis of PBC.
- Degree of elevation may corelate with ductopenia, disease progression, and may predict response to treatment.
- Elevated gamma-glutamyl transpeptidase is seen parallel with ALP rise.
- Serum Ig M levels may be elevated.
- Elevated serum transaminase levels may be seen reflecting degree of liver parenchyma inflammation and necrosis, however, are usually <5 ULN.
- Bilirubin is usually normal early in phases of the disease but elevated once disease progresses.
- Hypoalbuminemia, elevated INR, and thrombocytopenia are indicators of advancing disease.

Q. What is the role of Liver Biopsy in PBC and what are the staging systems?
Liver biopsy in PBC
Liver biopsy is not mandatory in the diagnosis of PBC.
Biopsy is indicated in cases of:

- AMA is negative or in low titer.
- Prominent hepatititic picture of elevation of transaminases.
- History of hepatotoxic drug intake.
- Suspicion of another concurrent pathology.
- Features of overlap with AIH.

Staging systems of PBC in liver biopsy
Histological hallmark of PBC is the presence of nonsuppurative cholangitis involving predominantly interlobular and septal bile ducts. Classically staging systems divide into four different stages.
Staging systems include

- Ludwig staging system
- Japanese (Nakanuma) staging system
- French staging system

Q. What Is AMA Negative PBC?
AMA Negative PBC

- Previously referred to as autoimmune cholangitis.
- Features of PBC with a negative AMA (Positivity for ANA and ASMA is seen in many cases).
- Constitutes 5% of the cases of PBC.
- Female predominance.
- Liver biopsy is a must for diagnosis.
- Differences in progression of disease are debatable with some studies reporting a more progressive disease.
- Similar response to PBC as AMA positive cases.

Q. Describe the role of UDCA in PBC
Ursodeoxycholic acid (UDCA)

- Widely studied and recommended by all society guidelines and recommended as first-line therapy.
- Mechanisms of action: Increase in hydrophilic bile acid profile, stimulation of bile secretion, immunomodulatory effects, and protection against cytokine-related injury.
- Dose: 13–15 mg/kg per day, either as a single oral daily dose or divided doses to improve tolerability.
- Side effects are minimal and include weight gain, hair loss, and GI disturbances like flatulence and diarrhea.
- Maximum benefit is early stages of the disease, although a survival benefit is demonstrable even in advanced disease.
- Stoppage of therapy leads to worsening liver functions thus mandating lifelong therapy.
- Safe during breastfeeding and lactation.
- Biochemical response at 1-year is a strong predictor of long-term prognosis in PBC.
- *Effects of UDCA in the natural history of PBC*
- The use of Ursodeoxycholic acid (UDCA) has an impact on modulation of the natural history of PBC. UDCA has been shown to significantly lower the histological progression to cirrhosis as well as prevent development of varices.

Criteria's for response to UDCA in PBC: Multiple criteria's have been used for assessment of response to UDCA at 1 year of treatment. Some of the commonly used criteria include:

Mayo criteria: ALP < 2 ULN
Paris I criteria: ALP < 3 ULN, AST < 2 times ULN, and Bilirubin < 1.0 mg/dl

Paris II criteria: ALP < 1.5 ULN, AST < 1.5 times ULN, and Bilirubin < 1.0 mg/dl
Spanish criteria: Reduction in ALP > 40% of baseline or to a normal value
Rotterdam criteria: Normalization of bilirubin and/or albumin, ALP, and platelets
Patients who fail to respond to these criteria have a higher probability of adverse
outcomes.

Q. What is the role of Obetecholic Acid (OCA) in PBC?

OCA is a highly selective oral Farnesoid-X-receptor semisynthetic agonist. It has
been shown to be efficacious in PBC based upon clinical trials.
   POISE trial: (Kowdley KV, et al. Hepatology. 2018;67(5):1890–902.)

- Nonresponders according to Toronto criteria.
- OCA showed evidence of biochemical efficacy with ALP > 1.67 ULN and/or
  bilirubin elevated < 2ULN.

Conditional approval in the following settings:

- In combination with UDCA for those with an inadequate response to UDCA.
- Monotherapy in those intolerants to UDCA.

Initial dose 5 mg; dose titration to 10 mg according to tolerability at 6 months.

Q. What are the other agents used in the management of PBC?
Other agents

- Budesonide: Currently not recommended.
- Fibric acid derivative: Bezafibrate: Although recent data suggests improvement
  in long-term prognosis as a combination therapy to UDCA currently not recommended (Corpechot C, et al New England Journal of Medicine.
  2018;378(23):2171–81).
- Under trial agents: Cilofexor, Seladelpar.

Q. How do you risk stratify and predict survival in PBC?
Risk stratification and survival models in PBC

- Transplant-free survival may be predicted by a biochemical response to UDCA
  as assessed Paris-1 (10-year transplant-free survival in responders >90%)
  Barcelona, and Toronto criteria.
- Mayo risk score is a widely used score that includes the following variables: age,
  total bilirubin, prothrombin time, albumin and presence/absence of peripheral
  edema, and response to diuretics. Mayo Risk Score > 4.1 serves as a threshold
  for HCC and variceal screening. Also used widely to estimate prognosis in liver
  transplant candidates.

- Elastography (LSM < 9.6 kPa vs. >9.6 kPa) has been used as a predictor for advanced disease.
- Continuous estimate mathematical models like UK-PBC and GLOBE risk scores accurately predict transplant-free survival at several time points and should be used to help better define the individual risk of development of complications of advanced liver disease.

Further Reading

European Association for the Study of the Liver. EASL Clinical Practice Guidelines: the diagnosis and management of patients with primary biliary cholangitis. J Hepatol. 2017;67(1):145–72.
Gulamhusein AF, Hirschfield GM. Primary biliary cholangitis: pathogenesis and therapeutic opportunities. Nat Rev Gastroenterol Hepatol. 2020;17(2):93–110.

Primary Sclerosing Cholangitis

2 Akash Roy, Prasanta Debnath, and Virendra Singh

Case Vignette A 38-year-old male presented with progressive jaundice for 20 days with associated itching, pale colored stools, and pain abdomen of 5 days duration. No history of complementary and alternative medicine use, surgical, or endoscopic biliary interventions in the past. There was a history of intermittent jaundice with pain abdomen (two episodes) in the last 1 year, which improved within 5–6 days of hospitalization with parenteral medication in a primary health center. He also complained of intermittent bloody diarrhea for the last 2 years, around 3–4 days in a month, with a bowel frequency of 2–3 episodes/day. He had no history of weight loss or loss of appetite. He had no history of any addictions and non-contributory family history. On examination, BMI was 20 kg/m^2, febrile, BP 110/70 mm of Hg, pulse rate of 100/min, icterus with scratch marks on the trunk and extremities, and shiny nails. The abdomen was soft with right upper quadrant tenderness; enlarged liver 3 cm below right costal margin. Spleen and gall bladder were not palpable.

Parameter	Values	Parameter	Values
Hemoglobin (g/dL)	11.2	INR	1.7
Platelet count (per mm^3)	188,000	HBsAg	Non-reactive
Total leukocyte count (per mm^3)	14,000	Anti-HCV	Non-reactive
Total bilirubin (Direct) (mg/dL)	12 (9.3)	ANA/ASMA/AMA	Negative
AST(U/L)	102	Na/K (mEq/dL)	132/4.3
ALT(U/L)	124	Urea(mg/dL)	32
ALP (N < 110)	391	Creatinine (mg/dL)	1

A. Roy · V. Singh (✉)
Department of Hepatology, Post Graduate Institute of Medical Education and Research, Chandigarh, Punjab, India

P. Debnath
Department of Gastroenterology, TNMC and BYL Nair Charitable Hospital, Mumbai, India

© The Author(s), under exclusive license to Springer Nature Singapore Pte Ltd. 2022
V. Singh, A. Roy (eds.), *Clinical Rounds in Hepatology*, https://doi.org/10.1007/978-981-16-8448-7_14

111

Parameter	Values	Parameter	Values
Albumin (g/dL)	3.2	IgM HAV	Negative
IgM HEV	Negative	pANCA	Positive

USG abdomen: Liver: 15 cm, raised echogenicity, short segment dilated supra-duodenal CBD 7 mm, no IHBRD; GB wall thickened; spleen and PV normal.

MRCP: Multifocal, short, annular strictures alternating with normal or slightly dilated segments producing a "beaded" pattern involving intra-hepatic bile duct, with dominant stricture involving CBD.

Ileo-colonoscopy: Pancolitis (Mayo Grade I).

Clinical Rounds

Q. What Is the Most Probable Diagnosis?

Ans: Primary Sclerosing Cholangitis (PSC) with associated Inflammatory Bowel Disease.

Q. How is the diagnosis of PSC made?

Ans: Patients with clinical profile suggestive of cholestatic jaundice with LFT showing raised ALP (R-ratio < 2) or LFT with mixed cholestatic-hepatitis profile (R-ratio between 2 and 5) or normal LFT with imaging suggestive of dilated CBD or intrahepatic biliary radicles, with cross-sectional imaging (MRCP) showing multifocal biliary strictures with segmental dilatation, in the absence of any other pathologies leading to same, are diagnosed as classic PSC. In some cases, ERCP can be used as a diagnostic modality where MRCP is inconclusive or is normal. Liver biopsy is required if ERCP is normal to look for **small duct PSC**.

Characteristic findings on liver biopsy:

I. Bile duct proliferation.
II. Peri-ductal fibrosis with typical "onion-skin" lesions.
III. Peri-ductal inflammation.
IV. Bile duct obliteration.

Q. Describe the cholangiographic changes in PSC
Cholangiographic changes in PSC (Amsterdam Classification):

Type	Intrahepatic	Extrahepatic
0	Normal	Normal
I	Multifocal change in duct contour; minimum dilatation	Slight irregularities of duct caliber; absence of stricture
II	Multifocal strictures; sac-like dilatations, reduced ductal arborization	Presence of segmental strictures

Type	Intrahepatic	Extrahepatic
III	With adequate filling pressure, only the central branches are opacified; severe narrowing with pruning present	Strictures involving the entire length of CBD
IV		Extremely irregular ductal contour; diverticulum-like outpouchings

Q. What is the role of autoantibodies in PSC?

There is an adjunct role for autoantibodies in the diagnosis of PSC. pANCA is non-specific, and mainly reflects the involvement of colon in patients presenting with cholestasis, without an underlying cause. Various autoantibodies that may be present in PSC are mentioned below, but are of uncertain value in diagnosis and prognostication:

- Anti-neutrophil cytoplasmic antibody (ANCA) in 50–80% of cases
- Anti-nuclear antibody (ANA) in 7–77%
- Anti-smooth muscle antibody (ASMA) in 13–20%
- Anti-endothelial cell antibody in 35%
- Anti-cardiolipin antibody (ACLA) in 4–66%
- Thyroperoxidase (anti-TPO) in 7–16%
- Thyroglobulin in 4%
- Rheumatoid factor (RF) in 15%

Q. What are the classical clinical features of PSC?

Ans: The natural history of PSC progresses through four sequential phases of clinical, biochemical, and histological abnormalities.

	Preclinical phase	Clinical phase	Symptomatic phase	Decompensated phase
Signs/ symptoms	Absent	Present	Signs and symptoms of chronic cholestasis and/or CLD. A small set of patients may present with recurrent bacterial cholangitis.	Present with complications of portal hypertension
LFT	Normal	Cholestatic LFT abnormalities present	Cholestatic LFT abnormalities present	Cholestatic LFT abnormalities present
Imaging	Classic biliary stricture may be present	MRCP/ERCP abnormalities—seen in 90–95%. (Around 45% of PSC patients are diagnosed in this phase)		

Modes of presentation:

A. Asymptomatic with abnormal LFT.
B. Known IBD patient on biochemical screening (cholestatic LFT abnormality).
C. Cholestatic symptoms like jaundice and pruritus.
D. Pain abdomen, jaundice, and fever in cholangitis.
E. Liver failure leading to jaundice.
F. Decompensated chronic liver disease with variceal bleeding and/or ascites.
G. Malignancy: Cholangiocarcinoma (CCA).

Presentation according to various symptoms

Symptoms	Prevalence (%)
Asymptomatic	15–44
Fatigue	43–75
Pruritus	25–59
Jaundice	30–69
Hepatomegaly	34–62
Pain abdomen	16–37
Splenomegaly	14–30
Increased pigmentation	25
Loss of weight	10–34
GI bleeding (variceal)	2–14
Ascites	2–10

Q. Discuss the differential diagnosis of the given case
Ans: Common causes to be considered on a case-by-case basis.
   Benign:

- **Choledocholithiasis**
- **Chronic pancreatitis**
- **Vascular:** Ischemic cholangiopathy, vasculitis, intraarterial chemotherapy, Portal cavernoma cholangiopathy.

   Infections: AIDS cholangiopathy, recurrent pyogenic cholangitis.
   Auto-inflammatory: IgG4 sclerosing cholangitis, Sarcoidosis, Eosinophilic cholangitis.
   Iatrogenic bile duct injury: Cholecystectomy (Open or Laparoscopic), Liver transplant (anastomotic stricture, non-anastomotic stricture).
   Malignancy: Cholangiocarcinoma, Pancreatic adenocarcinoma, Lymphoma, Secondaries from metastatic tumors.

Q. What are the clinical variants of PSC?

Ans:

Classic PSC: Involves both intrahepatic and extrahepatic bile ducts.

Small duct PSC: 5–10% at diagnosis.

PSC-AIH Overlap: 5–10% of PSC.

Other variants:

- Non-IBD PSC.
- Pediatric PSC (Autoimmune Sclerosing Cholangitis).

High-yield facts

- Isolated extra-hepatic duct involvement is seen in <5%.
- Concurrent IBD is seen in 60–80% of classic PSC. Prevalence of IBD among Asians with PSC 30–50%.
- PSC in UC: 2.3–4.6%, PSC in CD: 1.2–3.6%; In small duct PSC, CD > UC.
- PSC without IBD: Equal prevalence in males and females, older age at diagnosis, associated with good prognosis.
- Dominant stricture in PSC: 45–58% (during follow-up); Multiple strictures in 12%.
- Cholangiocarcinoma in PSC: 10–15% (AASLD).

Characteristics of IBD with PSC:

- Extensive colitis with pancolitis (Right-sided predominance of inflammatory activity).
- Sparing of rectum.
- Backwash ileitis more common.
- Milder disease activity.
- Higher risk of colorectal cancer.
- Higher risk of post-proctocolectomy pouchitis with IPAA.
- Higher risk of peristomal varices in patients with ileostomy.
    - Screening ileocolonoscopy with biopsy is recommended at the time of PSC diagnosis (*EASL, ESGE, ACG, AASLD*).
    - Yearly colonoscopic surveillance is advisable if IBD is diagnosed on either endoscopic or histologic examination.
    - In case of a negative diagnosis of IBD, next ileo-colonoscopy is advisable at 3–5 yearly interval, or whenever patients have bowel complaints, suggestive of IBD.

AASLD American association of study of liver disease, *EASL* European Association of Study of liver, *ACG* American College of Gastroentrology, *ESGE* European Society for Gastrointestinal Endoscopy

Q. What are the various prognostic indices and scores commonly used in PSC?

Ans:

Prognostic markers and indices:

Age: Increasing age is associated with poor prognosis.

Albumin: Inversely associated with prognosis, poor sensitivity in early disease.

ALP: Consistently associated with prognosis. However, fluctuating levels of ALP make it challenging for clinical application.

Small-duct PSC: Overall has a better prognosis compared to large duct PSC and is not associated with increased CCA risk.

Anti-GP2: Pancreatic autoantibody associated with poor liver transplant-free survival as well as having an association with cholangiocarcinoma.

Bilirubin: Persistently raised bilirubin for more than 3 months is associated with poor prognosis.

Dominant stricture: Associated with worse prognosis; however, endoscopic treatment has shown to improve liver transplant-free survival.

ELF test: Strong predictor of prognosis independent of the revised Mayo risk score.

IgG4 high PSC: Associated with shorter liver transplant-free survival.

Histological stage: As per the Nakanuma, Ishak, or Ludwig score.

Bile calprotectin: Parallels use of fecal calprotectin in IBD, underscoring the relationship between PSC and IBD.

Ultrasound spleen size > 12 cm: Associated with poor prognosis (LT, death, and decompensation).

Clinical scores:

Mayo score: Age, bilirubin, histological stage, hemoglobin, IBD.

King's College score: Age, histological stage, hepatomegaly, splenomegaly, ALP.

Multicenter model: Age, bilirubin, histological stage, splenomegaly.

Scandinavian model: Age, bilirubin, histological stage.

Revised Mayo score: Age, bilirubin, albumin, AST, variceal bleeding. **Most commonly used model.**

MELD score: Bilirubin, creatinine, INR.

Time-dependent score: Age at diagnosis, bilirubin, albumin.

PSC score: Age, albumin, bilirubin elevation >3 months, hepatomegaly, splenomegaly, dominant bile duct stricture, intra, and extrahepatic bile duct changes.

Q. How will you manage a case of PSC?

Ans: Holistic management approach:

Clinical diagnosis of PSC:

1. **Risk stratification:** The first step is risk stratification based on demographic variables, prognostic markers, and scores as well as presence/absence of dominant stricture.
2. **Stage of the disease**:
   (a) Fibrosis staging: Serum-based markers and elastography.
   (b) Cholangiopathy staging: MRCP, ERCP.
3. **Active management:** Involves addressing symptoms related to disease as well as associated complications (Cholangitis, Cirrhosis complications, Dominant strictures, Gall bladder polyps, CCA).
4. **Surveillance:**

(a) Symptoms and clinical evaluation: At least annually with MRCP if any changes.
(b) Gall bladder polyp: USG every 12 months.
(c) Rising LFTs: CA 19-9 and MRCP/CT.

Q. Define dominant stricture in PSC

Ans: A "dominant stricture" has been defined as stenosis with a diameter of 1.5 mm in the common bile duct or 1 mm in the hepatic duct (*AASLD*).

Dominant stricture at ERCP should be defined as stenosis with a diameter of ≤ 1.5 mm in the common bile duct and/or ≤ 1.0 mm in a hepatic duct within 2 cm of the main hepatic confluence (EASL/ESGE).

High yield points
The characteristic features of a stricture that suggests CCA are the ones that are disproportionately severe relative to others, concomitant biliary filling defects, and marked biliary dilatation (>2 cm for CBD, >1 cm for RHD/LHD, >5 mm for other intrahepatic ducts)
Decompression of biliary obstruction has been found to restrict further damage and can even lead to reversal of hepatic fibrosis
PSC patients attaining normalization or near normalization of ALP are found to have improved outcomes compared to those who do not
In patients with end-stage liver disease, only cholangitis is expected to improve with endoscopic intervention

Endoscopic Intervention in PSC:
Indications:

1. Clinically relevant or worsening symptoms (increasing jaundice, pruritus, or presence of cholangitis).
2. Rapidly increasing serum bilirubin and/or cholestatic enzymes (ALP/GGT), in patients with hilar or extrahepatic stricture(s).
3. New dominant stricture or progressing existing dominant stricture on MRCP (need to rule out CCA).

Endoscopic interventions in dominant strictures

- Consensus guidance recommends repeated endoscopic intervention (usually stricture dilatation ± stenting) of dominant biliary strictures in those with symptomatic disease.
- Endoscopic management of dominant biliary stricture is found to be beneficial in the management of jaundice, cholangitis, transplant-free, and overall survival in patients with PSC. Prospective study followed for 20 years, with repeated endoscopic therapy was shown to be associated with transplant-free survival of 81% at 5 years and 52% at 10 years after initial endoscopic therapy. Rate of CCA in that population was 6%.

• Endoscopic treatment should be performed with concomitant ductal sampling (brush cytology and/or endobiliary biopsy) of suspected significant strictures identified at MRC in PSC patients who present with symptoms likely to improve following endoscopic treatment.

Balloon dilation versus stent therapy:

Balloon dilatation in preference to stenting has been advised in European and American guidelines on the management of patients with PSC.

ESGE/EASL (2017) suggests that the choice between stenting and balloon dilation should be left to the endoscopist's discretion.

Some strictures do not dilate satisfactorily with balloon dilatation alone, and stent insertion is usually recommended in these cases.

Further Reading

Dyson JK. Primary sclerosing cholangitis. Lancet. 2018;391(10139):2547–59.

Chapman MH, et al. British Society of Gastroenterology and UK-PSC guidelines for the diagnosis and management of primary sclerosing cholangitis. Gut. 2019;68(8):1356–78.

European Society of Gastrointestinal Endoscopy et al. Role of endoscopy in primary sclerosing cholangitis: European Society of Gastrointestinal Endoscopy (ESGE) and European Association for the Study of the Liver (EASL) clinical guideline. J Hepatol 2017 66(6):1265–81.

Hepatocellular Carcinoma

15

Akash Roy, Virendra Singh, Harish Bhujade, and Naveen Kalra

Case Vignette

A 60-year-old man with background comorbidities of T2DM, essential hypertension, and dyslipidemia was diagnosed with NAFLD 6 years back. He was not on regular follow-up until recently when he did an ultrasonography which showed two space-occupying lesions measuring 3.4 cm and 2.9 cm, respectively. He was referred to hepatology services and was advised for a triple phase contrast CT scan. His labs and imaging findings are as follows:

Parameter	Values	Parameter	Values
Hemoglobin	11.2	INR	1.2
Platelet count	120	HBsAg	NR
Total leukocyte count	9000	Anti HCV	Neg
Total bilirubin (Direct)	2 (1.2)	Alpha-fetoprotein	12
AST	56	S Na/K	132/4.3
ALT	43	Urea/Creatinine	32/1
ALP	91	Albumin	3.3

Transient elastography: LSM 14.2 kPa CAP 286

TPCT W/A: Liver is irregular with nodular outline and caudate lobe hypertrophy. Two lesions measuring 3.4 × 2.2 cm and 3 × 3 cm in Seg VI and VII exhibit arterial enhancement and delayed phase washout. Portal vein is normal. There is no presence of any free fluid

A. Roy · V. Singh (✉)
Department of Hepatology, Post Graduate Institute of Medical Education and Research, Chandigarh, Punjab, India

H. Bhujade · N. Kalra
Department of Radiodiagnosis, Post Graduate Institute of Medical Education and Research, Chandigarh, Punjab, India

© The Author(s), under exclusive license to Springer Nature Singapore Pte Ltd. 2022
V. Singh, A. Roy (eds.), *Clinical Rounds in Hepatology*,
https://doi.org/10.1007/978-981-16-8448-7_15

Q. What is the probable diagnosis and how is the staging done and what are the recommended therapy specific to each stage?

In view of metabolic risk factors and possibility of non-alcoholic fatty liver disease (NAFLD) as well as biochemical and imaging evidence of cirrhosis, presence of SOL with characteristic imaging would suggest the possibility of Hepatocellular Carcinoma.

Multiple staging systems are used of which the most common is the Barcelona Clinic Liver Cancer System (BCLC System). In brief, the BCLC staging system is provided in Table 15.1.

Q. What is LI-RADS?

LI-RADS (Liver Imaging Reporting and Data System) is a classification system, which is used to estimate the likelihood of HCC in at-risk patients. It is validated only in patients with cirrhosis. The system provides a likelihood based on tumor characteristics including size, arterial phase enhancement, venous phase washout, capsule, and growth. Using these criteria, each lesion is classified into one of five major categories:

- LR-1: Definitely benign
- LR-2: Probably benign
- LR-3: Intermediate probability of malignancy
- LR-4 Probably HCC
- LR-5: Definitely HCC

Table 15.1 BCLC staging system for hepatocellular carcinoma

BCLC stage	Tumor characters	Extrahepatic spread	Child Class/ PS	Recommended therapy	Estimated survival
0 (Very early)	Single nodule <2 cm	Nil	CTP A PS 0	Curative Resection or liver transplantation (LT) depending upon portal pressure/ bilirubin	>5 years
A (Early)	Single or 2–3 nodules ≤3 cm	Nil	CTP A/B PS 0	Curative resection LT Ablation	
B (Intermediate)	Multinodular (unresectable)	Nil	CTP A/B PS 0	Palliative or downstaging to transplant by TACE, TARE	2 years
C (Advanced)	Extrahepatic spread	Portal vein or extrahepatic spread	CTP A/B PS 0–1	Systemic chemotherapy TACE/ TARE	8–13 months
D (Terminal)	End-stage liver function	Incurable and widespread disease	CTP C PS >2	Palliative therapy/ Best supportive care	3 months

Table 15.2 Classification systems in hepatocellular carcinoma

Classification system	Unique features
Alberta classification system (Canadian algorithm)	• Includes transarterial radioembolization (TARE) (yttrium) as a modality • Includes alpha-fetoprotein in algorithm • Provides for transplant beyond Milan criteria • Sorafenib restricted to Child Turcotte Pugh class A only
Hong Kong Liver Cancer System (HKLC)	• Predominantly derived from HBV-HCC cohort (Hepatitis B related HCC) • Early tumor: Single nodule ≤ 5 cm or ≤ 3 tumor nodule • Five stages I–V • Aggressive surgical resection
OKUDA	• First-staging system tumor and liver function • Tumor size (≤50% or >50% of the entire liver) • Predominantly a survival prediction system and limited role in guiding treatment decisions
Cancer of the Liver Italian Program (CLIP) score	• Prognostic scoring system • Includes alpha-fetoprotein-based stratification with cut-offs at 400 ng/dl
Model to Estimate Survival in Ambulatory HCC (MESIAH) Score	• Uses MELD as a measure to objectify prognosis • Predominantly as a supplement to BCLC to sub stratify each stage
AJCC-TNM staging system	• Pathological staging • Used for patients eligible for curative resection or liver transplant • No consideration of liver disease severity

Q. What are the other classification systems and what are their unique features?

Several classification systems exist which have attempted to stage and classify HCC for stratification and management purposes (Table 15.2).

Q. What are the Milan Criteria?

Based on a landmark study (Mazzaferro et al. NEJM 1996), a criterion was formulated which showed >90% recurrence-free survival at 4 years after liver transplant for HCC when lesions in the diseased liver satisfied the criteria and came to be known as the Milan criteria:

• Single tumor ≤5 cm or up to three tumors, each ≤3 cm
• No evidence of vascular invasion
• No extrahepatic spread (including regional lymph node involvement)

Q. What are the other criteria beyond Milan Criteria used for listing patients with HCC for Liver Transplant? (Table 15.3)

Table 15.3 Criteria beyond Milan criteria for transplant consideration in HCC

Criteria	Type of donor	Detailed criteria	Outcomes
UCSF (University of California San Francisco)	Cadaveric	Solitary tumor ≤6.5 cm or ≤3 tumors with largest ≤4.5 cm. Total tumor diameter ≤8 cm	5-year overall survival (OS), 72.4%
Up to Seven criteria	Cadaveric/ LDLT (both)	Seven: sum of tumor number and size of the largest tumor without microvascular invasion	5-year OS, 71.2%
Tokyo (5–5 rule)	LDLT (living donor liver transplant)	Maximum 5 tumors ≤5 cm	
Kyoto	LDLT	10 tumors ≤5 cm	
Hangzhou criteria	LDLT	Total tumor diameter ≤8 cm or <8 cm if grade I or II	5-year OS 70.7%
Asan	LDLT	≤6 tumors diameter ≤5 cm	
Samsung	LDLT/ Cadaveric	≤7 tumors, diameter ≤6 cm, AFP ≤ 1000 ng/ml	

Table 15.4 Common clinical presentation of HCC (adapted from Sleisenger and Fordtran's Gastrointestinal And Liver Disease, 10th edition)

Symptoms	Frequency(%)	Signs	Frequency (%)
Abdominal pain	59–95	Hepatomegaly	54–98
Weight loss	34–71	Ascites	35–61
Weakness	24–53	Fever	11–54
Abdominal swelling	28–43	Splenomegaly	27–42
Non-specific GI symptoms	25–28	Wasting	25–41
Jaundice	5–26	Hepatic bruit	6–25

Q. What are the common clinical presentations of HCC and what are the common sites of metastasis?

- Asymptomatic incidental
- Constitutional symptoms
- PUO (pyrexia of unknown origin)
- May develop decompensation in stable cirrhotics
- Abdominal mass
- Abdominal pain
- Jaundice
- Intraperitoneal bleed due to rupture (Table 15.4)

Site of extra hepatic metastasis in HCC: Lung > lymph node > bone > adrenal > peritoneum
Paraneoplastic manifestations in HCC

- Carcinoid syndrome
- Hypercalcemia
- Hypertension

- Hypertrophic osteoarthropathy
- Hypoglycemia
- Neuropathy
- Osteoporosis
- Polycythemia
- Polymyositis
- Porphyria
- Sexual changes—Precocity, gynecomastia, feminization
- Thyrotoxicosis
- Thrombophlebitis migrans
- Watery diarrhea syndrome

Q. What are the percutaneous strategies for tumor ablation strategies in HCC?

The ablative strategies that have been used in HCC are percutaneous ethanol injection (PEI), radiofrequency ablation (RFA), microwave ablation (MWA), cryoablation, and irreversible electroporation (Table 15.5).

The principle of RFA involves application of heat generated through high-frequency alternating current leading to coagulative necrosis and tumor death. RFA has been used as definitive therapy for early-stage HCC (BCLC 0 and BCLC A), with 5-year overall survival of up to 70% (Fig. 15.1).

Q. What are the Transarterial therapies in HCC? Mention briefly about the procedure for TACE

Transarterial therapies are modalities that serve as locoregional therapies in HCC, and include transarterial embolization (TAE), transarterial chemoembolization (TACE), and transarterial radioembolization (TARE) with yttrium-90 (Y90) microspheres. Common indications for transarterial therapies include BCLC-B patients or patients with multifocal or large tumors >2 cm.

According to the EASL guidelines, TACE is the recommended therapy for patients with BCLC-B stage HCC. TACE utilizes the principle of neo-angiogenesis in HCC by targeted intra-arterial administration of chemotherapy, followed by embolization of arterial feeders leading to cytotoxic and ischemic damage. The

Table 15.5 A brief comparison of the percutaneous procedures in the management of HCC

Radiofrequency ablation	Microwave ablation	Cryoablation	Irreversible electroporation
Can be monopolar or multipolar. Margins of ablation may be irregular in monopolar but multipolar RFA increases volume and predictability (margin) of ablation Zones **Limitations**: Thermal injury of adjacent structure Heat sink effect (near major vessels)	Higher and faster temperatures achieved in comparison to RFA More uniform zone of ablation **Limitations**: Heat sink effects	Easy monitoring of progression as imaging shows the ice ball formation **Limitations**: Cryoshock	Lower risk of thermal injury to adjacent vital structures Not affected by heat sink effect **Limitations**: Requirement of general anesthesia for the procedure

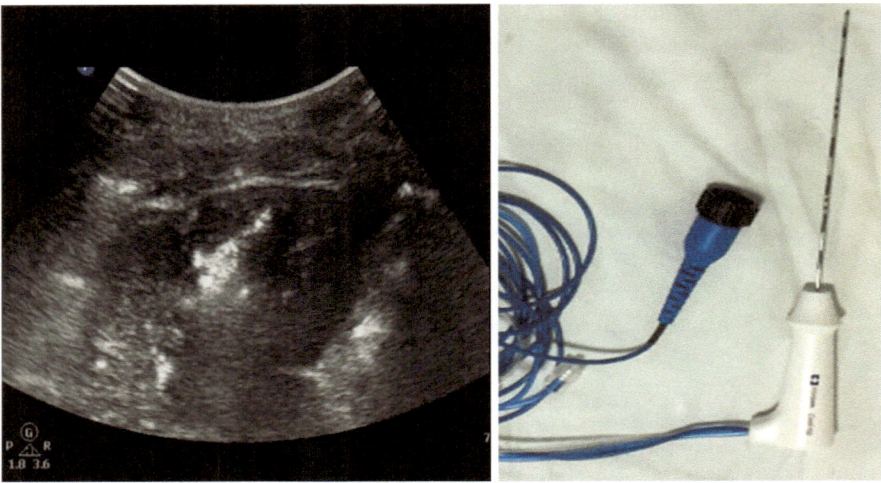

Fig. 15.1 Showing RFA probe (left) and a hepatocellular carcinoma treatment with RFA probe in situ (right)

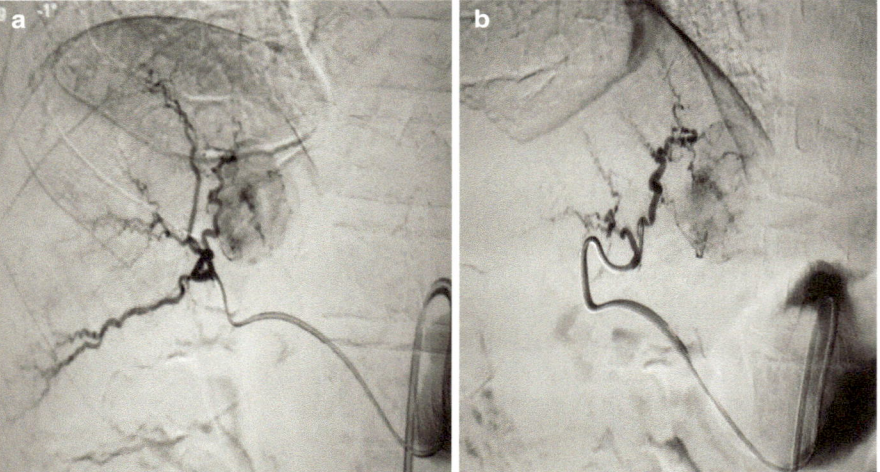

Fig. 15.2 Showing right hepatic angiogram (**a**) and selective angiogram (**b**) during the process of trans arterial chemoembolization

commonly used drugs used in TACE are doxorubicin and cisplatin. A modification of TACE is in the use of drug-eluting beads (DEB), which reduces systemic exposure to chemotherapy (Fig. 15.2).

Complications of TACE:

- Postembolization syndrome: Most common. It takes place due to direct effects of cytotoxic chemotherapy, cytokine release after tumor necrosis, and hypoxic

effects on normal liver parenchyma. Clinically it is manifested as liver enzyme abnormalities, fever, pain, and vomiting which is mostly self-limiting.
- Hepatic failure and decompensation.
- Abscesses.
- GI ulcerations.

The presence of portal vein thrombosis forms a relative contraindication to TACE. In such cases, TARE with Y90 has been proven to be safer.

Q. Describe the procedure of TARE and compare it with TACE
Indication

- Advanced unresectable HCC
- Bridge to liver transplant/downsizing

Procedure—can be divided into four stages:

- Patient preselection—identification of patient possibly eligible for this therapy.
- Patient selection—diagnostic angiography is performed to visualize the vascular anatomy and to identify and embolize any extrahepatic branch which could disperse the microspheres to non-target organs:
    - MAA (macroaggregated albumin) labelled with Tc99 are injected and SPECT/CT is done within 1 h of injection and lung shunt fraction (LSF) is calculated.
- Dose of Radionuclide to be used is calculated.
- Injection of Microspheres—1–2 weeks after planning session.
- Post Procedure—Bremsstrahlung SPECT/CT or Y90 PET-CT is done immediately post-procedure to verify that there are no Y90 microspheres in organs other than liver.

Dose modification based on LSF

- LSF <10%—no modification
- LSF 10–15%—reduce dose by 20%
- LSF 15–20%—reduce dose by 40%
- LSF >20%—contraindicated

Complications

- Liver Failure/Radiation-induced Liver Disease (RILD)
- Biliary complications
- Post embolization syndrome
- GI complications
- Radiation pneumonitis

Post-treatment protocol—No guidelines for timing of imaging after TARE. TPCT/MR 1 month after TARE and at 3-month intervals following the first treatment evaluation are the general recommendations.

Table 15.6 Characteristics of TARE and TACE in the management of HCC

TACE	TARE
Indications	
Stage: BCLC-B without vascular invasion	Stage: BCLC-B with lesions larger than 5 cm and or number of tumors >4
HCC with branch portal vein infiltration	HCC invading main portal vein or branch portal vein
Downstaging of HCC	Down staging
Contraindications	
HCC with main portal vein invasion	High shunt fraction >20
Extensive tumor replacing whole liver	Infiltrative tumor replacing whole liver
Severe cardiorespiratory disease	Severe cardiorespiratory disease
Bilirubin>3 mg/dl and or Creatinine >2	Bilirubin>3 mg/dl and/or Creatinine >2

Comparison between TARE and TACE: Meta-analysis data comparing the efficacy of TACE and TARE suggests that in cases of unresectable HCC, overall survival rates as well as 1-year progression-free survival to be are similar for TARE and TACE with TARE being associated with a higher probability of getting transplanted (Gardini et al. OncoTargets and Therapy 2018) (Table 15.6).

Q. What are the systemic therapy options available in the management of HCC?

Sorafenib: The mechanism of action of sorafenib involves multiple pathways which target growth factors including vascular endothelial growth factor receptors (VEGFR 1, 2, and 3), Raf MEK–ERK, and platelet-derived growth factor receptor-β (PDGFR-β). Based on the landmark SHARP trial it was shown that the median overall survival was 10.7 months in the sorafenib group in comparison to 7.9 months in the control group thus providing evidence for the use of sorafenib as the standard first-line therapy in advanced HCC (Llovet JM et al. New England Journal of Medicine 2008).

Side effects of sorafenib therapy: Diarrhea, hypertension, hand foot, and skin reactions (palmar-plantar erythrodysesthesia).

Lenvatinib: Lenvatinib is a newer molecule that has been found beneficial in the treatment of advanced HCC and targets multiple pathways including VEGFR, PDGFR, fibroblast growth factor receptors (FGFR), and KIT. In a recent trial, Lenvatinib led to a median survival time of 13.6 months which was non-inferior to 12.3 months with sorafenib 12.3 months (Kudo M et al. Lancet 2018).

Regorafenib: It is structurally as well as functionally similar to sorafenib and acts by inhibiting VEGFR and tyrosine kinase pathways. Based on the RESORCE trial regorafenib when used as a second-line therapy in patients who are progressors on sorafenib showed increased median survival and better disease control rates with regorafenib thus establishing its role as a second-line agent in advanced HCC (Bruix J et al. The Lancet. 2017).

Ramucirumab: It is a monoclonal antibody. Although the original trial with the drug did not meet its primary end points, subgroup of patients with alpha-fetoprotein >400 had both an improved median overall survival as well as progression-free survival with ramucirumab in comparison to placebo (Zhu AX et al. The Lancet Oncology 2019).

Q. What are the results and significance of the IMbrave 150 Trial in the landscape of HCC management?

The IMbrave 150 trial assessed the efficacy of combination of Atezolizumab (a selective PD-L1 inhibitor) and bevacizumab an anti-VEGF monoclonal antibody in the management of advanced unresectable HCC. It was an open-label trial with a 2:1 allocation ratio to receive atezolizumab (1200 mg) plus bevacizumab (15 mg/kg) every 3 weeks versus standard of care sorafenib. The 12-month overall survival was 67.2% with atezolizumab–bevacizumab and 54.6% with sorafenib. The median progression-free survival was 6.8 vs. 4.3 months. The most common adverse event noted in the trial was hypertension. This trial has provided the evidence for the first agent to outperform sorafenib in the first-line setting of unresectable advance HCC and is a landscape changer in the management options for HCC (Finn RS et al. New England Journal of Medicine 2020).

Q. What are the other emerging systemic options in the management of HCC?

- Immune checkpoint inhibitors in combination with locoregional therapy: Nivolumab plus TACE.
- Immune checkpoint inhibitors in combination with tyrosine kinase inhibitors: Lenvatinib plus pembrolizumab.

Further Reading

European Association For The Study Of The Liver. EASL clinical practice guidelines: management of hepatocellular carcinoma. J Hepatol. 2018;69(1):182–236.

Heimbach JK, Kulik LM, Finn RS, Sirlin CB, Abecassis MM, Roberts LR, Zhu AX, Murad MH, Marrero JA. AASLD guidelines for the treatment of hepatocellular carcinoma. Hepatology. 2018;67(1):358–80.

Kloeckner R, Galle PR, Bruix J. Local and regional therapies for hepatocellular carcinoma. Hepatology. 2021;73:137–49.

Hepatic Venous Outflow Tract Obstruction

16

Sahaj Rathi, Akash Roy, and Virendra Singh

Case Vignette

A 36-year-old male presented with a 1-month history of pain right upper abdomen and a 3-week history of abdominal distension. His family members noted yellowish discoloration of eyes lately. The patient had a history of vague pain off and on in her right upper abdomen for the past 2 years, for which she had been taking treatment from a local practitioner. There was no history of past jaundice, encephalopathy, or bleeding from any site.

Physical examination revealed pallor, scleral icterus, and pedal edema. The abdomen was uniformly distended with an everted umbilicus. Note was made of visible dilated tortuous vessels over the back. The liver was palpable 8 cm below costal margin in the midclavicular line. The spleen was palpable 6 cm below the costal margin. The presence of free fluid was evidenced by shifting dullness.

Laboratory investigations revealed the following:

Parameter	Values	Parameter	Values
Hemoglobin (gm/dL)	9.5	Na/K (mEq/L)	130/4.8
Platelet count (/µL)	78,000	Urea (mg/dL)	22
Total leukocyte count (/µL)	3000	Creatinine (mg/dL)	1.0
Bilirubin total/Direct (mg/dL)	4.4/2.7	INR	1.3
AST (IU/mL)	178	HBsAg	Neg
ALT (IU/mL)	90	Anti-HCV	Neg
ALP (IU/mL)	132	JAK-2	Neg
Albumin (g/dL)	3.2	Factor V Leiden	Neg

S. Rathi · A. Roy · V. Singh (✉)
Department of Hepatology, Post Graduate Institute of Medical Education and Research, Chandigarh, Punjab, India
e-mail: rathi.sahaj@pgimer.edu.in

© The Author(s), under exclusive license to Springer Nature Singapore Pte Ltd. 2022
V. Singh, A. Roy (eds.), *Clinical Rounds in Hepatology*,
https://doi.org/10.1007/978-981-16-8448-7_16

An abdominal ultrasound showed an enlarged liver (span 19 cm), with irregular outline. The right and middle hepatic veins were visualized, but their confluence with the IVC was not visualized. The left hepatic vein was not visualized. There were multiple comma-shaped veno-venous collaterals within the liver parenchyma. The spleen measured 17 cm. Portal vein diameter was 13 mm, and there was a moderate amount of free fluid.

Q. What is the most probable diagnosis based on the given vignette?
A: Hepatic Venous Outflow Tract Obstruction/Budd Chiari Syndrome.

Q. What Is HVOTO/BCS?
Primary BCS/HVOTO is defined as the obstruction of the hepatic venous outflow anywhere from the level of the small hepatic veins to the cavo-atrial junction in the absence of intracardiac or pericardial obstruction. The obstruction of hepatic venous outflow due to compression by metastases, infiltrative liver diseases, or liver abscesses is referred to as secondary BCS.

Q. How do patients with HVOTO/BCS present?
The clinical presentation of BCS is quite variable. The age at presentation is different in different geographical regions, suggesting a difference in the etiopathological pattern of disease. Data from the East shows an early onset, often in the second or third decade, with a male predominance. However, Western data indicates a presentation in a fourth-fifth decade with a slight female preponderance.

An acute, complete occlusion of the hepatic venous outflow may lead to a catastrophic presentation with severe pain, ascites, jaundice, and coagulopathy. However, in most cases, the presentation is more gradual. A history of right upper abdominal pain is usually present (over 60%). Ascites (83%) and hepatomegaly (67%) are seen in most patients. Up to 15–20% of patients may be asymptomatic and detected incidentally.

The presence of dilated, tortuous veins over the flank or back indicate obstruction of the IVC, and are highly suggestive of HVOTO/BCS in the appropriate clinical setting. The direction of flow in these vessels is from below upward, as these vessels shunt blood from IVC drainage territories to the SVC.

Q. Describe the pathophysiological alterations in BCS/HVOTO?
The underlying pathophysiology in BCS/HVOTO hepatic parenchymal congestion is due to poor hepatic venous outflow. This may be a consequence of blocked hepatic veins, obstruction at the level of intrahepatic IVC, or a combination of the two. In most cases, thrombosis of the hepatic veins is the likely initial event, which may later organize into a fibrotic occlusion. There is a considerable heterogeneity in the epidemiological, clinical as well as pathological features of patients with BCS/HVOTO. This is due mainly to varied predisposing factors, location and extent of obstruction, and the acuity of occlusion.

The rapidity and extent of occlusion determine the clinical presentation—patients with acute, complete occlusion of all three hepatic veins present with an acute, fulminant hepatitis. However, most patients usually have a more sedate course. The progressive, asynchronous, and differential occlusion of hepatic veins leads to alternative drainage of congested parenchyma into adjoining venous territories, leading to the development of intraparenchymal and subcapsular veno-venous collaterals. As the caudate lobe has independent drainage into the IVC, it remains unaffected by the occlusion of hepatic veins, which leads to its hypertrophy. Other areas of hepatic parenchyma which manage to achieve effective drainage through collaterals develop hypertrophy, leading to a heterogeneous vascular and parenchymal distribution. The IVC may be compressed by the hypertrophied caudate lobe, further compromising venous outflow. This ongoing congestion leads to hepatocyte ischemia and necrosis, sinusoidal capillarization, endothelial dysfunction, and stellate cell activation, ultimately leading to progressive fibrosis. The necrosis and following fibrosis are predominantly around the central vein, giving rise to a venocentric pattern of collagen deposition, known as "reverse lobulation" (Fig. 16.1).

Q. What are the predisposing factors for the development of HVOTO/BCS?
The presence of hypercoagulable states is considered a strong risk factor for the development of this disease. However, the data again is quite heterogenous with a wide geographic divide. While Western studies have identified an underlying prothrombotic state in a majority of cases (~80%), estimates of identifiable prothrombotic state among Eastern studies vary between 10 and 70% cases. Among these, myeloproliferative neoplasms and acquired thrombophilic disorders like factor V Leiden mutation are the most common. Other factors include Protein C, Protein S, Antithrombin III deficiency, APLA syndrome, Behcet's disease, and paroxysmal nocturnal hemoglobinuria.

Q. When would you suspect BCS/HVOTO?
The diagnosis of BCS/HVOTO required a high degree of clinical suspicion. Features of chronic liver disease in patients with an enlarged liver, especially in the younger age groups, should raise suspicion. History of right upper quadrant pain in this clinical context further favors BCS/HVOTO.

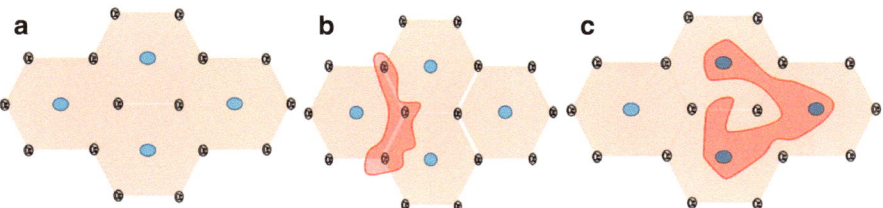

Fig. 16.1 (**a**) Normal Hepatic lobule, with central vein (Pale blue) at the center, and Portal triads (Black outline ovals with red, white, and green circles representing hepatic artery, portal vein, and bile duct). (**b**) Porta based lobule, with hepatocyte damage along the portal tracts (Red area). (**c**) Reverse lobulation, with hepatocyte damage along the central veins (Red area)

Q. How is the diagnosis of BCS/HVOTO established?

The diagnosis of BCS/HVOTO requires non-visualization, thrombosis, or obstruction of at least two hepatic veins. Doppler ultrasound is usually the first-line investigation in the diagnosis. Presence of hepatic parenchymal or subcapsular veno-venous collaterals (comma-shaped collaterals) is a pathognomonic feature. These collaterals attempt to drain the parenchyma of the territory of the blocked vein into the IVC directly or via accessory veins. The liver is usually enlarged, variegated in appearance, with a hypertrophied caudate lobe. The margins are often irregular due to underlying fibrosis as well as the presence of regenerative nodules. The intrahepatic IVC is frequently narrowed due to compression from a hypertrophied caudate lobe. Spectral doppler of the hepatic veins shows loss of the normal phasic variation of flow, however, this feature may also be seen in cirrhosis and highly steatotic livers.

Contrast-enhanced CT or MR venography performs better at characterizing the intra- and extrahepatic collaterals. BCS/HVOTO often leads to a characteristic pattern of enhancement in the post-contrast sequences—the hypertrophied caudate lobe and other areas close to the IVC take up contrast faster, and wash out faster than the more peripheral areas, creating a differential pattern of enhancement (flip-flop enhancement, Fig. 16.2). This occurs as the caudate lobe and the regions closer to IVC are more effectively drained, and therefore less congested. The lack of contrast opacification of the hepatic veins does not always mean thrombosis, as contrast may not have entered the hepatic veins due to congestion—this should always be confirmed using doppler ultrasound.

Cross-sectional imaging also helps to identify and characterize focal lesions in the liver, which are common among these patients. However, it is often difficult to differentiate regenerative nodules from hepatocellular carcinoma in these patients as both show arterial enhancement, and up to 30% regenerative nodules may show washout. The presence of an elevated AFP, size >3 cm, and the presence of a capsule in the delayed phase makes the diagnosis of HCC more likely.

Q. What is the pathogenesis of ascites in HVOTO/BCS?

The impediment of hepatic venous outflow leads to an increase in the hydrostatic pressure within the sinusoids. This leads to increased exudation of tissue fluid

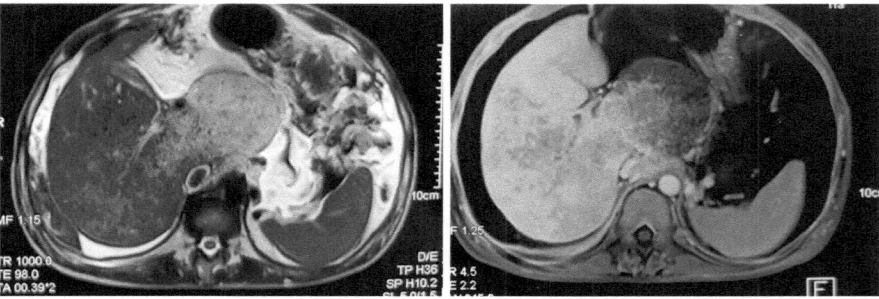

Fig. 16.2 MRI images in a patient with Budd Chiari showing differential enhancement

from the sinusoids into the interstitium. As the sinusoids are fenestrated with wide intercellular spaces, proteins are easily able to go across the sinusoids, leading to a protein-rich tissue fluid within the interstitium. In the early stages, this increased protein-rich interstitial fluid is taken away by the lymphatics. However, as the severity of disease progresses, this fluid overwhelms the capacity of lymphatics, and oozes out of the liver capsule, leading to high protein ascites.

The sinusoidal congestion also leads to hepatocellular necroinflammation, endothelial damage, and stellate cell activation. As a result, there is deposition of collagen within the perisinusoidal space of Disse, and reduction in the intercellular spaces in the sinusoidal lining ("capillarization" of the sinusoid). Thus, the proteins which could previously flow freely through the sinusoidal gaps are now restricted to the sinusoidal space, and only protein poor fluid goes into the interstitium, and as a result of overwhelmed lymphatics, into the peritoneal cavity. This leads to low protein ascites in the advanced stages of Budd-Chiari syndrome.

Q. What are the fallacies in assessment of severity of liver disease in BCS/HVOTO?

Assessment of severity of liver disease is complex in these patients, as many of the manifestations of advanced liver disease are seen early on. Varices, ascites, jaundice, can all be seen even before the onset of cirrhosis as features of a congested liver. Irregular liver outline on imaging may be due to regenerating nodules, and mimic cirrhosis. Albumin may be low due to parenchymal synthetic dysfunction or as a negative acute phase reactant. Noninvasive assessment of liver fibrosis by elastographic techniques may be fallacious too, as increased liver stiffness may be a consequence of congestion as well as fibrosis. However, the transition of high protein ascites to low protein ascites is a proxy for sinusoidal capillarization and development of perisinusoidal fibrosis, and may indicate development of cirrhosis. Other complications of liver cell failure like development of encephalopathy and hepatorenal syndrome also indicate the development of advanced liver disease.

Multiple prognostic scores have been used to risk-stratify patients with BCS/HVOTO. These include CTP and MELD Score, Clichy BCS index, Rotterdam score, AIIMS-HVOTO score, etc. However, while these scores are a good way to compare data among studies, their external validity and implication on individual patient decisions are quite limited.

Q. How would you manage a patient with BCS/HVOTO?

Management of BCS/HVOTO is complex and requires multidisciplinary involvement. Due to the heterogeneity of disease across geographic regions and the paucity of well-designed, randomized controlled trials, most treatment protocols are institutional and expert consensus based.

The focus of therapy is to decongest the liver, and prevent further progression of the thrombus. This may be achieved by medical management with anticoagulation, thrombolysis, reopening of the hepatic outflow with angioplasty/stenting. If recanalization of physiological outflow is not possible, creating a portosystemic shunt to bypass the liver may be required. If the patient fails this management, or has poor liver reserve, liver transplantation is the ultimate option.

Medical Management

Patients with BCS often have underlying prothrombotic states. Lifelong anticoagulation is considered preventive against progression of disease, and is recommended by most consensus guidelines. However, this recommendation is weak, as there have been no controlled studies to study the effectiveness of this approach. This fact is even more pertinent when managing patients in the East, where underlying thrombophilic states are not as well documented. It is unclear if patients with BCS/HVOTO with fibrotic/membranous outflow obstructions would benefit from anticoagulation. Therefore, this decision should merit a discussion weighing the pros and cons in each individual patient.

Decongestive Measures

Hepatic decongestion may be achieved by alleviating the obstruction to hepatic venous outflow, or by shunting the blood from the portal to systemic circulation.

1. Targeting hepatic outflow obstruction

    Nearly a third of patients with BCS/HVOTO have short segment stenosis of hepatic veins or IVC. In such cases, the priority should be to alleviate the outflow obstruction in order to achieve physiologic flow. This may be achieved by angioplasty and/or stenting of the hepatic veins and/or IVC.

    A transjugular or transfemoral approach may provide access to the hepatic veins for decompressive procedures. However, in some cases where technical limitations prevent entry into the hepatic veins, percutaneous access may be used.

    It is important to understand the pressure gradients before planning these procedures, and an IVC venography with pressure measurements across the intrahepatic IVC is important. If the pressure gradient across a stenotic segment of IVC is >8–10 mmHg, the obstruction of IVC is considered significant (Fig. 16.3).

2. Portosystemic shunting

    If physiological antegrade flow cannot be achieved with the above procedures, decongestion of the liver is attempted by creating a portosystemic shunt. This may be achieved radiologically or surgically.

    If a substantial hepatic vein is visualized, a standard TIPS procedure connecting the hepatic and the portal veins may help decompress the liver. However, often none of the hepatic veins are visualized. In such cases, it may be reasonable to create a new shunt between the IVC and the portal vein. This short, side-to-side portocaval shunt is known as a Direct Intrahepatic Porto-Systemic Shunt. Most of these procedures are technically challenging in the setting of BCS/HOVTO, and should be attempted preferably at expert centers.

    Surgical creation of a portosystemic shunt was previously common, but is used less with the advent of advanced interventional radiological techniques. However, these may be a rescue in case a radiological creation of TIPS or DIPS

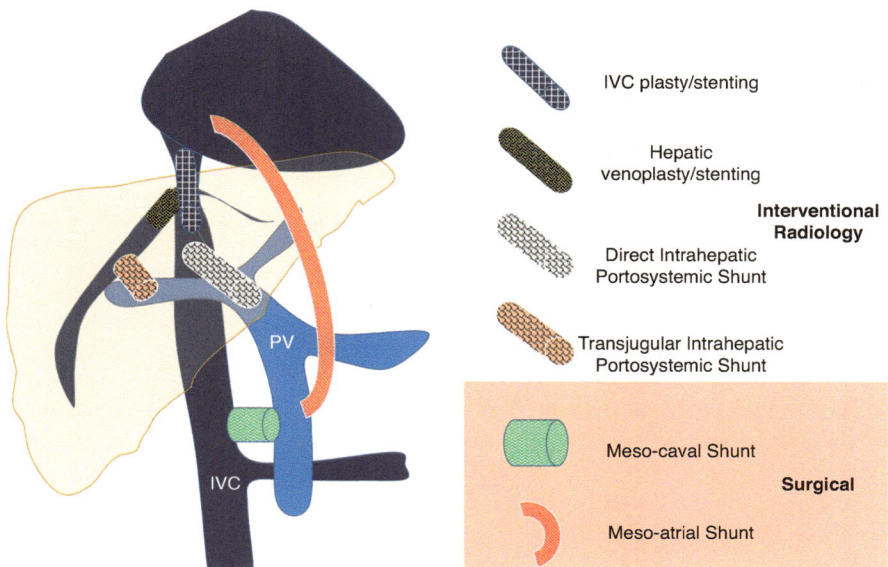

Fig. 16.3 Schematic of decongestive options for BCS/HVOTO

is not technically feasible. A mesocaval shunt connects the superior mesenteric vein to the IVC in a side-to-side manner. In case of severe IVC stenosis, a meso-atrial shunt can bypass the stenotic segment and connect the mesenteric vein directly to the right atrium with an artificial vascular graft, achieving effective decongestion. However, the success and patency rates of surgical shunts vary widely with centers, and are associated with higher risk of postoperative complications, especially in the setting of a poor liver reserve. Moreover, these may make future liver transplantation more complicated. Therefore, a detailed inter-disciplinary discussion is required for every individual patient before embarking upon any decongestive procedure (Fig. 16.3).

Liver Transplantation

Liver transplantation is the ultimate option in patients with poor liver reserve, or those who fail to improve after anticoagulation and/or decongestion. The posttransplant outcomes are good, with 5-year survival rates up to 80%. It is important to identify and characterize prothrombotic states before transplantation, so that appropriate anticoagulation may be instituted in the posttransplant period. Underlying myeloproliferative neoplasms are known to increase vascular complications, but do not affect survival. Previously placed TIPS/hepatic vein stents do not seem to adversely affect the outcomes of liver transplantation.

What are the risks for hepatocellular carcinoma in BCS?

Hepatocellular carcinoma has been frequently reported in patients with BCS with a prevalence similar to that in chronic viral hepatitis-associated cirrhosis although wide variations exist in published literature. The diagnostic approach to

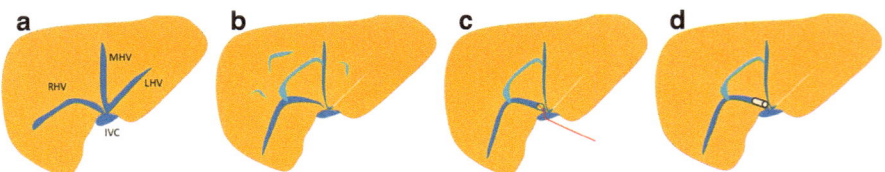

Fig. 16.4 (**a**) Representative cross-sectional anatomy of normal hepatic veins draining into IVC. (**b**) Schematic for index patient—The Left Hepatic Vein (LHV) is thready. The Middle (MHV) and the Right (RHV) hepatic veins are narrowed at their confluence with the IVC. There are multiple comma-shaped veno-venous collaterals, with one connecting MHV and RHV. (**c**) A balloon being for venoplasty of RHV. (**d**) A stent was placed within the RHV. The MHV is also draining into the RHV through the large collateral

focal liver lesions in the context of BCS is challenging and requires expertise in differentiating nodular lesions from true HCC. The risk factors that have been associated with development of HCC in BCS are presence of underlying cirrhosis, location and length of vascular obstruction, and presence of a long-standing hepatic venous outflow obstruction.

Case Vignette: Followup

The patient was further evaluated with an MR venography and the vascular anatomy was delineated. He had a stenotic confluence of the right and the middle hepatic veins with the IVC, and a large intrahepatic collateral connecting the middle and the right hepatic vein. The inferior venacava was narrowed, but had a pressure gradient of 5 mmHg. He underwent a venoplasty and stenting of the right hepatic vein, and was started on anticoagulation. This led to improvement of his pain, liver functions, and ascites (Fig. 16.4).

Further Reading

Qi X. Budd Chiari syndrome. 1st ed. Singapore: Springer; 2019.

Northup PG, Garcia-Pagan JC, Garcia-Tsao G, et al. Vascular liver disorders, portal vein thrombosis, and procedural bleeding in patients with liver disease: 2020 practice guidance by the American Association for the Study of Liver Diseases. Hepatology. 2021;73:367–413.

Valla DC. Budd–Chiari syndrome/hepatic venous outflow tract obstruction. Hepatol Int. 2018;12(Suppl 1):168–80.

Surender Singh, Akash Roy, and Virendra Singh

Q. Define Sarcopenia and enumerate the diagnostic criteria for Sarcopenia?
The term sarcopenia is defined as "a progressive and generalized skeletal muscle disorder associated with an increased likelihood of adverse outcomes including falls, fractures, physical disability, and mortality." The European working group on sarcopenia in older people (EWGSOP) provides the criteria for both diagnosis and staging of sarcopenia, which are enumerated in Tables 17.1 and 17.2.

Q.What are the modalities for evaluating sarcopenia?
- **Mid-arm muscle circumference (MAMC)**: Ready to use bedside tool, which is widely available. However, it has low reproducibility, and its observations are affected by subcutaneous adipose tissue loss.

Table 17.1 EWGSOP diagnostic criteria for sarcopenia

Presence of criteria number 1 plus either criterion number 2 or 3
1. Low muscle mass
2. Low muscle strength
3. Low physical performance

Table 17.2 EWGSOP staging of sarcopenia

Stage	Muscle mass	Strength	Physical performance
Pre-sarcopenia	Decreased		
Sarcopenia	Decreased	Decreased	Decreased
Severe sarcopenia	Decreased	Decreased	Decreased

S. Singh · A. Roy · V. Singh (✉)
Department of Hepatology, Post Graduate Institute of Medical Education and Research, Chandigarh, Punjab, India

© The Author(s), under exclusive license to Springer Nature Singapore Pte Ltd. 2022
V. Singh, A. Roy (eds.), *Clinical Rounds in Hepatology*,
https://doi.org/10.1007/978-981-16-8448-7_17

- **Bioelectrical impedance analysis (BIA)**: Noninvasive and easy-to-use modality. However, results are affected by fluid retention, diuretic use, food intake, and physical activity.
- **Dual-energy X-ray absorptiometry (DEXA)**: Widely available modality. However, its principle limitation is its lack of applicability in the presence of edema.
- **Ultrasound (thigh muscle thickness)**: Noninvasive and easy to use modality which can be used as a bedside tool. However, accurate cut-offs and reproducibility need to be validated.
- **Cross-sectional imaging (CT/MRI)**: Currently, considered as the gold standard for sarcopenia assessment. Precision is the key advantage with these modalities as observations are not influenced by presence of ascites and edema. The primary limitations lie in the concern for radiation exposure, especially when repeated measurements are required.

Q. What are the reported prevalence of sarcopenia in cirrhosis, and how does it affect prognosis?

Sarcopenia has been variably reported in cirrhosis, with prevalence ranging from 31 to 70%, depending on the different indices used for defining sarcopenia. Montano-Loza et al. assessed the presence of sarcopenia in 112 patients with cirrhosis using CT scan at L3 vertebra to calculate the skeletal muscle index (SMI). SMI includes the total cross-sectional areas of the psoas, erector spinae, quadratus lumborum, transversus abdominis, external and internal obliques, and rectus abdominis (normalized to height). The cut-offs of SMI ≤ 38.5 cm^2/m^2 for women and ≤ 52.4 cm^2/m^2 for men were considered appropriate for the diagnosis of sarcopenia according to this study. When sarcopenia was correlated to outcomes, it was identified as an independent predictor of mortality (Montano-Loza AJ et al. Clinical gastroentrology and hepatology 2012).

In a recent study, patients with cirrhosis listed for liver transplant were assessed for sarcopenia using CT scan to calculate SMI at L3 vertebral level. Using a cut-off of <50 cm^2/m^2 for males and <39 cm^2/m^2 for females, sarcopenia was present in 50% men and 33% of women. This study also reinforced the fact that sarcopenia was associated with increased wait-list mortality in cirrhosis ($p < 0.001$) (Carey EJ et al. Liver Transplantation 2017).

Q. What do you mean by the term sarcopenic obesity in cirrhosis?

Sarcopenic obesity refers to a state in patients with cirrhosis who are obese and are sarcopenic. It has been most commonly defined in terms of CT scan-based height corrected SMI, and for assessment of overweight and obesity as a BMI of ≥ 25 or ≥ 30 kg/m^2.

Defining criteria's for sarcopenic obesity in cirrhosis
Obesity (one of the following definitions)

- Body mass index ≥ 30 kg/m^2(Asian: ≥ 25 kg/m^2)
- A percentage of fat mass $\geq 28\%$ in males and $\geq 40\%$ in females
- Central obesity (one of the following):

- A waist circumference '102 cm in men and '88 cm in women (Asian: Waist circumference '90 cm in males and '80 cm in females).
- A visceral fat area ≥100 cm² on abdominal CT.

Sarcopenia (criterion "a" plus either "b" or "c")

(a) Decreased muscle mass (one of the following definitions should be present):
   - Appendicular skeletal muscle mass (ASM)/squared height (m²)
   - Skeletal muscle mass index (SMI)
(b) Decreased muscle strength
(c) Low physical performance

Q. What is meant by the term myosteatosis?
Myosteatosis is a state in which there is a pathological accumulation of fat in skeletal muscle. The fat accumulation can be either within the muscular fibers (intramyocellular fat) or within the muscle fascia (intermuscular fat). Myosteatosis quantification can be done by muscle biopsy, CT or magnetic resonance imaging, and magnetic resonance spectroscopy (MRS). The radiodensity of skeletal muscle measured by CT correlates well with intramyocellular fat content measured by MRS and skeletal muscle fat content determined by percutaneous muscle biopsy. Myosteatosis has been labeled as an emerging prognostic factor in cirrhosis. It is reported in more than 50% of patients with cirrhosis evaluated for liver transplantation and is associated with an independently higher risk of hepatic encephalopathy.

Q. What is meant by the term frailty?
Frailty is a concept that has its primary origin in geriatric literature. Unlike sarcopenia, which specifically connotes to the loss of muscle mass and function, frailty is a deterioration in the physiological reserve leading to an increased vulnerability to health stressors with subsequent physical dependency and multiple adverse outcomes, including death.

Q. What are the tools used in the measurement of Frailty?
Multiple assessment tools have been developed which identify patients who are frail or are at risk for frailty. These include:

- **Activities of daily living (ADL)**
- **Instrumental activities of daily living (IADL)**
- **Karnofsky Performance Scale (KPS)**
- **Clinical Frailty Scale (CFS)**
- **Braden Scale**
- **Fried Frailty Phenotype (FFP)**: This is the most commonly used assessment tool for frailty. It was devised with a primary focus on the geriatric population to identify those with functional decline. It categorized frailty depending on five characteristics: weight loss, exhaustion, weakness, slow walking speed, and decreased physical activity.

- **Handgrip strength (HGS)and gait speed test (GST)** are easy to use bedside tests to screen for frailty.
- **Short Physical Performance Battery (SPPB)**: Includes repeated chair stands, balance testing, and a 4-m walk.

Q. What is Liver Frailty Index (LFI)?

Liver Frailty Index (LFI) is a frailty assessment tool in patients with cirrhosis. It combines hand grip strength, chair stands, and balance to assess frailty in cirrhosis. It is seen to be independent of the degree of liver dysfunction, and it outperforms classical frailty assessment Fried Frailty Phenotype (FFP) and Short Physical Performance Battery (SPPB). Additionally, LFI is also readily reproducible and practical in daily clinical use. Stratification based upon LFI:

- **Robust LFI < 3.2**
- **Pre-frail 3.2 ≤ LFI < 4.5**
- **Frail LFI ≥ 4.5**.

Q. Mention the role of myostatin and ammonia in the pathogenesis of Sarcopenia

Myostatin is a growth factor often referred to as a myokine, which in simple terms is produced from the myocyte and acts on muscle cells to inhibit its proliferation. It belongs to the transforming growth factor-beta family and serves as a negative regulator of satellite cells that control myocyte proliferation. Ammonia concentrations are thought to be directly proportional to myostatin upregulation. Besides myostatin upregulation, ammonia also stimulates the activation of the ubiquitin-proteasome pathway, proteophagy, and mitochondrial oxidative damage.

Q. What are the prognostic implications of Sarcopenia and Frailty on transplant waitlist mortality?

MELD-sarcopenia score: The MELD-sarcopenia score was developed to incorporate sarcopenia assessed by CT scan muscle mass measurements and expressed as a dichotomous variable. The MELD-sarcopenia score's ability to predict waitlist mortality was significantly improved with the addition of sarcopenia as a component (Montano-Loza AJ et al. Clinical and translational gastroentrology 2015).

Similarly, the **Liver Frailty Index (LFI)**, when used in combination with MELD-Na, showed a better predictive ability of 3-month mortality and also allowed for a 19% reclassification of deaths/delisting in waitlisted patients (Lai JC et al. Hepatology 2017).

Q. What are the proposed measures for the improvement of Sarcopenia and Frailty in cirrhosis?

The principal approaches toward the improvement of sarcopenia in cirrhosis for optimization prior to transplant include:

- Nutrition: High-protein/high-calorie diet, late evening snacks, BCAA supplementation.
- Exercise: 30- to 60-min sessions of combined aerobic and resistance training with the goal to achieve 150+ min/week of moderate intensity exercise. The minimum duration of any exercise intervention program has been shown to be at least 3 months (Chodzko-Zajko WJ et al. Medicine and science in sports and exercise 2009).
- Testosterone supplementation.
- L-ornithine L-aspartate and rifaximin.

Further Reading

Carey EJ, et al. A North American expert opinion statement on sarcopenia in liver transplantation. Hepatology. 2019;70(5):1816–29.

Buchard B, et al. Assessment of malnutrition, sarcopenia and frailty in patients with cirrhosis: which tools should we use in clinical practice? Nutrients. 2020;12(1):186.

Sinclair M, et al. Sarcopenia in cirrhosis–aetiology, implications and potential therapeutic interventions. Aliment Pharmacol Ther. 2016;43(7):765–77.

Yogendra Kumar, Akash Roy, and Virendra Singh

Q. How do you assess surgical risk in cirrhosis?
The consensus on 30-day mortality after surgery in cirrhosis based upon Child Turcotte Pugh score is as follows:

- CTP-A 10%
- CTP-B 30%
- CTP-C of 76–82%

Factors affecting adverse outcomes after surgery include:

- Liver injury due to anesthetic or hypotension during surgery.
- Shifts in fluid balance.
- Delayed wound healing.
- Bleeding tendency.

Role of MELD: MELD has been shown to be a good predictor of 30-day mortality after surgery. It shows a linear relationship with mortality, with mortality rising by 1% for each MELD point below 20 and by 2% for higher MELD scores. In 2007, the largest study to predict mortality in cirrhotics undergoing surgery using the MELD scores was conducted. The median survival based on MELD score is shown in table. This study's results were used to formulate the Mayo Clinic Model, which gives the Mayo Risk Score (MRS), which comprises **Age, ASA class, bilirubin, INR, creatinine, and etiology of cirrhosis**. The study was based upon a review of case records of 700 patients undergoing cardiac, orthopedic, or gastrointestinal surgeries (except Cholecystectomy) from 1980 to 2004. It showed increased mortality at 90 days

Y. Kumar · A. Roy · V. Singh (✉)
Department of Hepatology, Post Graduate Institute of Medical Education and Research, Chandigarh, Punjab, India

postoperatively compared with ambulatory patients. However, the study is limited by the fact that the majority of patients had low baseline MELD score (Median MELD-8) with platelet count >60000/μl and INR < 1.5 (Teh SH et al. Gastroenterology, 2007).

Other factors that may affect outcomes after surgery include:

- Hyponatremia
- Low serum albumin
- Older age
- Serum creatinine
- Emergency versus elective surgery
- Type of surgery—abdominal/GI surgery possibly has the worst outcomes

Q. What Is the VOCAL-Penn Risk Assessment Score?

Recently researchers from the University of Pennsylvania have devised a new score new score called the VOCAL-penn (Veteran's Outcome and Cost Associated with Liver Disease), which incorporates the following parameters:

- Age
- Albumin
- Bilirubin
- Platelet count
- Presence or absence of NAFLD (non alcoholic fatty liver disease)
- BMI > 30
- ASA score
- Type of surgery
- Emergency of surgery

The performance of the score was found to be superior to MELD, MELD-Na, CTP, and Mayo Risk Score at predicting 0, 90, and 180-day postoperative mortality.

Q. How to manage pruritus in Cholestatic Liver Disease?

Ans: Stepwise approach for the treatment of pruritus in liver diseases:

Approach	Drug	Dose	Interactions/precautions
1st line	Cholestyramine	4–16 g/day	Interference with intestinal absorption and hence 4-h interval with administration of concomitant medications like ursodeoxycholic acid
2nd line	Rifampicin	150–600 mg/day	Enzyme induction leading to altered drug metabolism and potential risk of hepatotoxicity
3rd line	Bezafibrate[a]	200–400 mg/day	Nephrotoxicity Myopathy and rhabdomyolysis
4th line	Naltrexone	25–50 mg/day	To be started at lower doses and careful titration

Approach	Drug	Dose	Interactions/precautions
5th line	Sertraline	75–100 mg/day	QTc prolongation and potential for malignant neuroleptic syndrome
6th line	**Experimental approaches**	Gabapentin Phenobarbital UVB light Albumin dialysis Nasobiliary drainage	Administration recommended only in specialized centers

[a]**FITCH Trial**: Bezafibrate in cholestatic liver disease and sclerosing cholangitis with moderate to severe pruritus. A total of 45% of the patients experienced a 50% or higher reduction in itch intensity within 3 weeks of treatment (de Vries et al., Hepatology, 2019)

Q. What is portal cavernoma cholangiopathy (PCC)?

PCC is defined as abnormalities in the extrahepatic biliary system, including the cystic duct and gallbladder with or without abnormalities in the 1st- and 2nd-generation biliary ducts in a patient with portal cavernoma.

All of the following criteria should be satisfied for making the diagnosis:

- Presence of a portal cavernoma
- Typical cholangiographic changes on ERCP or MRCP
- Absence of other causes of these biliary changes

Q. What are the cholangiographic abnormalities seen in PCC?

The characteristic cholangiographic abnormalities include:

- Extrinsic impressions/indentations
- Shallow impressions/indentations
- Irregular ductal contour
- Stricture
- Filling defects
- Bile duct angulation
- Upstream dilatation
- Ectasia

Q. What are the venous plexuses around the biliary tract?

Two venous plexuses drain the biliary tract, which includes a fine reticular epicholedochal **venous plexus of Saint** on the wall of the bile duct, which drains into the paracholedochal **venous plexus of Petren** (also called marginal veins or parabiliary venous system), which in turn is connected to the posterior superior pancreaticoduodenal vein, gastrocolic trunk, right gastric vein, and superior mesenteric vein inferiorly as well as intrahepatic portal vein branches superiorly.

Q. What is the pathophysiology of biliary changes in PCC?

The development of biliary changes in PCC is due to two components :

(a) Reversible component (55%): These occur due to compression of the bile ducts by engorged collaterals and tend to reverse after shunt surgery.
(b) Fixed component (45%): Likely due to ischemic changes in the bile duct.

Q. What is the natural history of PCC?

Usually, a diagnosis of EHPVO when associated with PCC usually antedates symptomatic PCC by 8–10 years. The natural history of PCC can be divided into four stages:

1. **Preclinical**: Presence of portal cavernoma but no PCC with normal liver biochemistry and no symptoms of PCC.
2. **Asymptomatic**: Early changes on cholangiography with normal or abnormal liver biochemistry but no symptoms.
3. **Symptomatic**: Advanced changes on cholangiography with abnormal liver biochemistry and presence of symptoms without complications.
4. **Complicated**: Presence of liver dysfunction or fibrosis, extensive biliary changes like multifocal strictures or calculi above strictures.

Q. What are the diagnostic modalities used in PCC?

1. USG with color doppler is the initial imaging modality for suspected cases of PCC.
2. MRCP with MR portovenography:
   (a) Serves as a comprehensive noninvasive technique.
   (b) As accurate as ERCP in delineating biliary changes.
   (c) Demonstrates relationship of biliary changes with collaterals.
   (d) Presence of shuntable vein can be ascertained.
   (e) Helps to distinguish between bile duct varices and common bile duct stones.
3. EUS is helpful in delineating the type of choledochal collaterals:
   (a) **Paracholedochal**: Varices at a distance from the fibromuscular layer.
   (b) **Pericholedochal**: Large varices (>1 mm) which lie outside and adjacent to the fibromuscular layer.
   (c) **Epicholedochal**: Small varices (<1 mm) which lie outside and adjacent to the fibro-muscular layer.
   (d) **Intracholedochal**:
       (i) Varices at <1 mm distance from stent or stone.
       (ii) Varices with CBD wall on both sides.
4. **ERCP**
   Traditionally been the gold standard for diagnosis of PCC.
   Due to its invasive nature, risk of complications, and need for sequential imaging, it has now been replaced by noninvasive radiological modalities for diagnosis. Classification systems include:

Chandra classification:

Type I: Involvement of extrahepatic ducts only.

Type II: Involvement of intrahepatic bile ducts only.

Type IIIa: Extrahepatic bile duct with unilateral intrahepatic bile duct involvement.

Type IIIb: Extrahepatic bile duct with bilateral intrahepatic bile duct involvement.

Llop classification:

Grade I: Irregularities or angulations of the biliary tree.

Grade II: Indentations or strictures without upstream biliary dilation.

Grade III: Strictures with upstream biliary dilation.

*Dilatation is defined as ductal diameter of >7 mm for extrahepatic duct and/or >4 mm for intrahepatic ducts.

5. **IDUS and cholangioscopy**

Q. What are the management strategies in PCC?

Asymptomatic patient: No treatment is advocated. Patients with PCC and other associated abnormalities like deranged LFT without symptoms should be regarded as having asymptomatic PCC, and are not candidates for endoscopic therapy.

Approach to symptomatic PCC:

Phased manner of symptomatic PCC management:

First phase:

Sphincterotomy and biliary drainage, with CBD stone removal if present.

Further management:

- Repeated plastic stent exchange or placement of removable covered metal stents.
- Repeated stent exchanges over short periods of time (3–5 years) may occasionally result in the resolution of stenosis.
- Concomitant use of ursodeoxycholic acid (UDCA) may be beneficial.

Portal decompression surgery:

- Can be used as first phase of therapy in patients in whom endoscopic intervention is not required (e.g., patient with isolated stenosis of CBD and with a shuntable vein).
- Usually used as second phase of therapy in symptomatic PCC.
- Involves portal decompression surgery by proximal splenorenal shunt or TIPSS.
- Shunt procedures result in regression of changes of cholangiopathy in 62–88% of patients.
- 25–30% of patients will require further intervention for PCC after a successful shunt procedure.
- Nonsurgical candidates: Absent shuntable vein (5–30%) or advanced liver dysfunction.

Third phase of therapy: Patients who remain symptomatic despite shunt procedure either due to blockage of shunt or due to persistent obstruction despite patent shunt may be candidates for second-stage biliary drainage surgery like hepaticojejunostomy or choledochoduodenostomy.

Liver transplantation: Secondary biliary cirrhosis is the only accepted indication for liver transplantation in patients with complicated PCC.

Q. Describe in brief AIDS cholangiopathy

- Stricture formation of the biliary tract due to opportunistic infections leading to biliary obstruction and cholestatic liver damage.
- Prevalence—Variably reported (26–46% in Pre-HAART era).
- **Risk factors**
  - CD4 < 100.
- **Etiology**
  - *Cryptosporidium parvum* is the commonest pathogen associated with AIDS cholangiopathy—(20–57%).
  - Cytomegalovirus: Up to 20% of cases are due to vascular injury.
  - *Microsporidia*: 10%
- **Symptoms**—Variable presentations ranging from asymptomatic to severe right upper quadrant pain associated gastrointestinal symptoms:
  - Fever and jaundice are less commonly seen
  - Substantial weight loss is commonly seen
  - Pruritus is remarkably uncommon
- **Diagnosis**—MRCP and ERCP have the same sensitivity for diagnosis of AIDS cholangiopathy:
  - Papillary stenosis (PS) is the commonest reported finding.
  - In 2/3rd papillary stenosis (PS) is present either alone or in combination with intrahepatic ductal dilatation and multifocal intrahepatic biliary strictures with alternating normal segments or saccular dilatations.
  - 20% of cases may have a characteristic beaded appearance.
  - 6–15% have 1–3 cm segmental extrahepatic biliary stricture with or without intrahepatic involvement.
- **Management**
  - Symptomatic treatment: Opioids and neural plexus blocks for abdominal pain.
  - Treatment of opportunistic infection is usually ineffective.
  - Use of UDCA has been shown to improve abdominal pain and normalization of liver function abnormalities after sphincterotomy for papillary stenosis.
  - The best treatment is the restoration of immune function using HAART or switching to second-line HAART if there is resistance.
  - Endoscopic sphincterotomy.

Q. What are the diagnostic criteria for Ig-G4 cholangiopathy?
Diagnostic items

1. **Biliary tract imaging** reveals diffuse or segmental narrowing of the intrahepatic and/or extra-hepatic bile duct associated with the thickening of the bile duct wall.
2. **Hematological examination** shows elevated serum IgG4 concentrations ($\geq$135 mg/dl).
3. **Associated disease**: Coexistence of autoimmune pancreatitis, IgG4-related dacryoadenitis/sialadenitis, or IgG4-related retroperitoneal fibrosis.
4. **Histopathological examination** shows:
   (a) Marked lymphocytic and plasmacyte infiltration and fibrosis.
   (b) Infiltration of IgG4-positive plasma cells: >10 IgG4-positive plasma cells/HPF.
   (c) Storiform fibrosis.
   (d) Obliterative phlebitis.

Optional: Effectiveness of steroid therapy
Definite diagnosis: (1) + (3) or (1) + (2) + (4) a, b or (4) a, b, c **or** (4) a, b, d
Probable diagnosis: (1) + (2) + Optional criteria
Possible diagnosis: (1) + (2)
It is necessary to exclude PSC, malignant diseases such as pancreatic or biliary cancers, and secondary sclerosing cholangitis. When it is difficult to differentiate from malignant conditions, a patient must not be treated with empirical steroid therapy but should be referred to a specialized medical facility.

Q. How do you distinguish between IgG4-SC and Primary Sclerosing Cholangitis (PSC)?

Category	Feature	Details
Type 2 IgG4 SC vs. PSC		
Clinical	IBD	Seen in 75% of PSC and whereas 5% in IgG4-SC,
	Age and gender	• Usually presents before 40 years in PSC and >50 years in IgG-4 SC • Males predominance is seen in both entities (1.5:1 in PSC & 7:1 in IgG4-SC)
Lab	pANCA	40 vs. <10%
	sIgG4 >1.4 g/l	In 9–18% of PSC and 65–80% of IgG4-SC
	sIgG4 >5.6 g/l	100% specificity for IgG4-SC
	sIgG1:IgG4 ratio	95% specificity of ratio >0.24 for IgG4-SC versus PSC-high IgG4 (sIgG4 1.4–2.8 g/l)
Imaging	Cholangiogram	• Beaded or pruned-tree appearance and short band-like strictures in PSC • Long continuous strictures with prestenotic dilatation, involvement of the distal common bile duct and hilar or intrahepatic cholangiopathy in IgG4-SC
	CT scan	• Evidence of other organ involvement, especially pancreatic involvement (92%) in IgG4-SC

Category	Feature	Details
Histology	Morphology	• Onion-skin fibrosis and periportal sclerosis in PSC • Classical features in IgG4
	IgG4+:IgG+ plasma cell ratio	• In PSC-high IgG4, ratio <40% • In IgG4-SC, IgG4+plasma cells >10/HPF (biopsy) or >50/HPF (resection), ratio >40%
Treatment	Steroids	• Response in IgG4-SC with biochemical and radiological improvement at 4 weeks in two-thirds of patients with IgG4-SC and almost 100% of patients with AIP • No response in PSC; however, variable response in overlap syndromes and in patients with PSC-high IgG4

Q. What are the management options of patients with IgG-4 SC?
Management principles in IgG-4 SC include initiation of remission and further maintenance therapy

Induction of remission:

1. Oral prednisone: (0.6–1 mg/kg) for 3 weeks and then taper over 3–6 months.
2. Rituximab (1 g iv infusion at week 0 and week 2).

Maintenance therapy:

1. Low dose glucocorticoids.
2. Disease-modifying drugs: Agents like Azathioprine, mycophenolate mofetil, 6-Mercaptopurine, and Tacrolimus have been used for remission maintenance.
3. Rituximab: 1 g infusion therapy administered every 6 months.

Q. Enumerate the Swansea Criteria for diagnosis of Acute Fatty Liver of Pregnancy (AFLP)

AFLP is a rare ((1: 20,000 pregnancies) but dreaded complication in pregnancy). It presents as an emergency with a high risk to both mother and fetus. The pathogenesis of AFLP is centered upon fetal defects in the mitochondrial beta-oxidation chain. Due to the defects, there is an accumulation of unmetabolized long-chain fatty acids in the fetal circulation initially and then into the maternal circulation, which ultimately is deposited in the maternal liver which triggers liver dysfunction. The most commonly observed defect is due to mutations leading to deficiency in the long-chain 3-hydroxyacyl coenzyme A dehydrogenase (LCHAD) enzyme. The clinical criteria for the diagnosis are given by the Swansea Criteria:

Six or more of the following features in the absence of other identified etiology:

• Vomiting
• Abdominal pain
• Polydipsia/polyuria
• Encephalopathy

- Bilirubin (>14 µmol/l)
- Hypoglycemia (<4 mmol/l)
- Leukocytosis (>11 × 10⁶/l)
- Elevated uric acid (>340 µmol/l)
- Elevated ammonia (>42 IU/l)
- Ascites or bright liver on ultrasonography
- Elevated transaminases (>42 IU/l)
- Renal impairment (creatinine>150 µmol/l)
- Coagulopathy (PT > 14 s or APTT > 34 s)
- Microvesicular steatosis on biopsy

Q.What is the concept of "Rebalanced Hemostasis" in Cirrhosis?
Historically, it was believed that cirrhosis is a state of "auto-anticoagulation" and is always associated with bleeding tendencies. However, evolving literature has suggested that there is a balance of both procoagulants and anticoagulants in cirrhosis.
   Procoagulant changes in cirrhosis

- ↓ Protein C and protein S
- ↓ Anti-thrombin
- ↑Factor VIII
- ↑ Von Willebrand Factor

Anticoagulant changes in cirrhosis

- ↑ Fibrinolysis
- ↓ Factors II, VII, IX, and X
- Thrombocytopenia
- ↓ Platelet function

Further Reading

Culver EL, et al. IgG4-related hepatobiliary disease: an overview. Nat Rev Gastroenterol Hepatol. 2016;13(10):601–12.
Dhiman RK, et al. Portal cavernoma cholangiopathy: consensus statement of a working party of the Indian national association for study of the liver. JCEH. 2014;4(Suppl 1):S2–S14.

Keisham Amarjit, Akash Roy, and Virendra Singh

Q. What are the indications for Liver Transplantation evaluation, and what is the role of the MELD Score in transplant prioritization?

Liver transplantation is based on the principle that it should be considered in any patient with advanced liver disease in whom transplantation would extend life expectancy beyond what is expected as per the natural history of the disease. The indications for an evaluation for liver transplantation include:

1. Acute liver failure
2. Acute on chronic liver failure
3. Decompensated cirrhosis and its complications (ascites, variceal hemorrhage, hepatic encephalopathy)
4. Hepatocellular carcinoma
5. Metabolic disorders of the liver (alpha-one anti-trypsin deficiency, familial amyloidosis, primary hyperoxaluria, glycogen storage disorders, hemochromatosis)
6. Systemic complications of chronic liver disease (hepatopulmonary syndrome, porto-pulmonary hypertension)

The timing of offering liver transplantation is crucial as offering LT early may have limited benefits. Before 2002, the allocation was based on the CTP score, which has multiple limitations. In 2002, the MELD (Model for end-stage liver disease) score was introduced to objectify transplant prioritization. Since in patients who have a MELD ≤ 14 transplantation does not lead to better survival as compared to the natural course of the disease, a cut-off of MELD ≥ 15 has been taken as an indication to listing for transplant with certain exceptions.

K. Amarjit · A. Roy · V. Singh (✉)
Department of Hepatology, Post Graduate Institute of Medical Education and Research, Chandigarh, Punjab, India

© The Author(s), under exclusive license to Springer Nature Singapore Pte Ltd. 2022
V. Singh, A. Roy (eds.), *Clinical Rounds in Hepatology*, https://doi.org/10.1007/978-981-16-8448-7_19

MELD Exceptions
Manifestations of cirrhosis

- Refractory ascites.
- Hepatopulmonary syndrome: The presence of severe HPS is associated with increased mortality and affected individuals should undergo expedited LT evaluation.
- Porto-pulmonary hypertension: LT can be offered to potential recipients with POPH, which responds to medical therapy with a mean pulmonary artery pressure of ≤35 mmHg.
- Intractable pruritus non-responsive to medical therapy.

Miscellaneous liver diseases

- Budd-Chiari syndrome
- Familial amyloidotic polyneuropathy
- Cystic fibrosis
- Hereditary hemorrhagic telangiectasia
- Polycystic liver disease
- Primary oxaluria
- Recurrent cholangitis
- Uncommon metabolic disease

Malignancy

- Cholangiocarcinoma
- Hepatocellular carcinoma

Q. What are the contraindications to Liver Transplantation?
Although the practice of LT is ever-evolving and previously unexplored areas are being explored, the general contraindications to LT include:

- Severe cardiac or pulmonary disease
- Ongoing alcohol or illicit substance abuse
- Hepatocellular carcinoma with metastatic spread
- Uncontrolled sepsis
- An anatomic abnormality that precludes liver transplantation
- Extrahepatic malignancy
- Hemangiosarcoma
- Persistent noncompliance
- Lack of adequate social support system

Q. What are Extended Criteria Donor (ECD) Graft and Criteria for Marginal Graft?

ECD graft is a graft with suboptimal characteristics which may be associated with poor graft function. A marginal liver donor is defined as:

- Donor aged >65 years
- ICU stay with ventilation >7 days
- BMI >30
- Steatosis of the liver >40%
- Serum sodium >165 mmol/L
- Transaminases: ALT >105 U/L, AST >90 U/L
- Serum bilirubin >3 mg/dL

Q. What are the principles of Volumetric Assessment of a donor in a Living Donor Liver Transplant (LDLT)?

In cases of LDLT, the primary safety concern is to ensure the adequate residual volume of the donor's liver. The donor must have at least 30% of residual liver volume after hepatectomy, and the graft-to-recipient weight ratio (in g/kg) must be at least 0.8–1.0. This ratio approximately amounts to around 45–50% of the standard recipient liver volume and is deemed adequate to meet the graft's metabolic requirements. A specific condition called Small for Size Syndrome (SFSS) can develop when the graft is small, resulting in graft dysfunction.

Q. Briefly describe Primary Non-function and Hepatic Artery Thrombosis Following Liver Transplantation

Primary non-function (PNF): Seen in 5% of overall transplants and presents liver cell failure features. Factors associated with the development of PNF include graft steatosis >30%, history of prolonged hospitalization, increased use of inotropes before transplantation, prolonged cold ischemia time (CIT), and donation after cardiac death (DCD) donors. Additionally, seen more commonly in patients undergoing re-transplantation. Management of PNF is re-transplantation, and patients are listed as a medical urgency if they have the following features:

AST ≥3000 and one or both of the following within 7 days of transplant:

- INR ≥2.5
- Arterial pH ≤7.3 or venous pH of 7.25
- lactate ≥4 mmol/L

Hepatic artery thrombosis (HAT): Seen in 3–9% of overall transplants. The incidence of HAT is usually higher with complex arterial reconstructions. Presentation is either detected as an incidental finding on serial doppler ultrasound posttransplant or with elevated aminotransferase levels. Frequently seen in conjunction with biliary complications. Management involves revascularization or re-transplantation.

Q. How is acute Cellular Rejection (ACR) after Liver Transplant classified?

Acute cellular rejection (ACR) is seen in 15–25% of LT recipients and has a favorable prognosis with early immunosuppression optimization. It occurs as an inflammation of the donor graft and affects interlobular bile ducts and the vascular endothelium.

Classification

A. **Based on timing after LT**
   • Early ACR in the first 3–6 months after LT.
   • Late ACR after 3–6 months from LT
B. **Histological severity classification (Banff classification)**
   • The histological features suggestive of ACR include mixed inflammatory infiltrate, bile duct inflammation/damage, and subendothelial inflammation. These parameters are individually graded on a scale of 0–3 (mild, moderate, severe) to give the composite Rejection Activity Index (RAI).

Q. What are the options in the management of ACR?

The principle of ACR management include optimization of the immunosuppression.

Strategies include:

• Pulse Methylprednisolone: 500 mg–1 g for 1–3 days.
• Addition of immunosuppressive drugs with the ongoing regimen (mTor inhibitors, MMF, Tacrolimus).
• Thymoglobulin: 1.5 mg/kg/day for 5–7 days.
• Anti-IL-2Rα antibodies.
• Anti-CD3 monoclonal antibody (OKT3).

Q. What are the risk factors for chronic rejection, and what are the principles of it's management?

• Any previous episode of acute cellular rejection.
• Previous episode of moderate or severe acute rejection.
• Donor age ≥40 years.
• Transplantation for primary disease as primary biliary cirrhosis and autoimmune hepatitis.
• Recipient age ≤30 years.
• CMV (cytomegalovirus) IgG-positive donor into a negative recipient or CMV infection.

The principles of managing chronic rejection are either optimization of ongoing immunosuppression regimen or re-transplantation if there is non-response to the former. Since chronic rejection pathogenesis involves a multifactorial causation, treatment is generally difficult. Some studies have tried mTOR inhibitors (Sirolimus or Everolimus) as add-on immunosuppression which has shown variable impact (Nishida S et al. Transplant Proc., 2001).

Q. How are infections in a transplant recipient classified according to time since transplant?

0–30 days

The most common infections are surgical site infections, pneumonia, catheter-related bloodstream infections (CRBSI), catheter-associated urinary tract infections (CAUTI), and *Clostridium difficile*.

31–180 days

In addition to the infections seen during the first month, CMV disease commonly occurs once prophylaxis has been discontinued (especially in donor positive, recipient negative (D+R− cases). Other opportunistic infections include *Aspergillus* and *Cryptococcus*, *Nocardia*, and tuberculosis.

>180 days

The risk of infection gradually reduces post 6–12 months after liver transplantation. In cases of suspicious infections, the common differentials that need to be excluded include CMV, *Cryptococcus*, tuberculosis, endemic fungi (e.g., histoplasmosis), and EBV-related PTLD.

Q. What is the 6-Month abstinence rule in Liver Transplantation?

The 6-month abstinence rule refers to an arbitrary time interval of 6 months of abstinence from alcohol that has been recommended prior to liver transplantation in patients with alcohol-related liver disease. The time period is, however, arbitrary and is based upon the concept that abstinence allows assessment of disease progression/regression after alcohol consumption is stopped, allows time for psychological preparation and also serves as a surrogate marker for predicting potential relapse in patients with alcohol-related liver disease. This concept has however been challenged on the grounds of high mortality without transplantation, especially in patients with alcoholic hepatitis as well as poor predictive capacity for posttransplantation alcohol relapse. In a landmark study, it was shown that patients with severe AH (corticosteroid nonresponders) who underwent early LT had a significantly better survival rate as compared to those who did not (Mathurin P et al. Early liver transplantation for severe alcoholic hepatitis. NEJM, 2011).

Q. Describe in brief the ACCELERATE-AH Trial for transplantation in Alcoholic Hepatitis?

The trial evaluated the role of early liver transplantation (LT) (without a mandated period of sobriety) for patients with severe alcoholic hepatitis (Lee BP et al. Gastroenterology, 2018). The key features of the trial were:

- Retrospective study design ($N = 147$)
- The median duration of abstinence before LT was 55 days
- 54% received corticosteroids for AH
- Median Lille score of 0.82, MELD-Na score of 39

- 1 year survival %: 94%
- 3-year survival: 84%

Q. Briefly summarize the Evidence for Liver Transplantation in Acute on Chronic Liver Failure

Authors	Number of patients	Results	Comments
Levesque et al. 2017	140	70% survival at 1 year as compared to 92% in those without ACLF	ACLF-3 had the worst outcomes 17/30 (56%) mortality at 1 year in ACLF 3
Artru et al. 2017	73	83.9% survival at 1 year with baseline ACLF grade 3	7.9% survival in patients not transplanted All patients had complications and longer hospital stay
Moon DB et al. 2017	189 ACLF 136 (non ACLF)	76.8% survival at 1 year and 70.5% at 5 years	ACLF patients had a longer stay in ICU
Yadav et al. 2017	52	88.5% survival at 90 days post-transplant	Non-LT ($n = 68$) had 32.4% survival at 6 months

Q. What are the milan Criteria?

Based on a landmark study (Mazzaferro et al. NEJM, 1996), a criterion was formulated which showed >90% recurrence-free survival at 4 years after liver transplant for HCC when lesions in the diseased liver satisfied the criteria and came to be known as the Milan criteria:

- Single tumor ≤5 cm or up to three tumors, each ≤3 cm
- No evidence of vascular invasion
- No extrahepatic spread (including regional lymph node involvement)

Q.What Are the Other Criteria Beyond Milan Criteria Used for Listing Patients with HCC for Liver Transplant?

Criteria	Type of donor	Detailed criteria	Outcomes
UCSF	Cadaveric	Solitary tumor ≤6.5 cm or ≤3 tumors with largest ≤4.5 cm. Total tumor diameter ≤8 cm	5-year overall survival of 72.4%
Up to Seven criteria	Cadaveric/ LDLT (both)	Sum of tumor number and size of the largest tumor without microvascular invasion up to 7 cm	5-year overall survival of 71.2%

Criteria	Type of donor	Detailed criteria	Outcomes
Tokyo (5–5 rule)	LDLT	Up to 5 tumors ≤5 cm	
Kyoto	LDLT	Up to 10 tumors ≤5 cm	
Hangzhou criteria	LDLT	Total tumor diameter ≤8 cm or <8 cm if grade I or II	5-year OS 70.7%
Asan	LDLT	≤6 tumors diameter ≤5 cm	
Samsung	LDLT/ Cadaveric	≤7 tumors, diameter ≤6 cm, AFP ≤1000 ng/mL	

LDLT Living donor liver transplantation, *AFP* alpha-fetoprotein

Q. What Is the Mayo Clinic protocol for LT in Cholangiocarcinoma (CCA)?

Initial experiences of orthotropic liver transplantation for unresectable CCA were extremely poor because of the frequent recurrence and a 5-year survival rate of 5–15%. However, a cohort of long-term survivors prompted the development of a protocol at the University of Nebraska and Mayo Clinic for neoadjuvant chemoradiation followed by OLT in highly selected patients with early stage, unresectable hilar CCA. (De Vreede I et al. Liver Transpl., 2000).

Key features of the protocol are:

- Preoperative management: 5-Fluorouracil (5-FU) used in combination with external beam radiation therapy (EBRT) over 4 weeks followed by four sessions of brachytherapy. Post the initial session patients are put on oral Capecitabine. Close to the expected time of transplantation and at least 2 weeks after brachytherapy, all patients undergo a pretransplant staging exploratory laparotomy to evaluate for metastatic disease. Regional lymph nodes are biopsied during the procedure, even if they seem benign.
- The first reported series of patients transplanted according to this protocol 45% tumor-free survival with a median follow-up of 7.5 years.

Further Reading

Murray KF, et al. AASLD practice guidelines: evaluation of the patient for liver transplantation. Hepatology. 2005;41(6):1407–32.

Part II

Biliary and Pancreatic Disorders

20

U. V. U. Vamsidhar Reddy, Akash Roy, and Virendra Singh

Case Vignette A 45-year-old female was admitted with right upper quadrant pain, nausea, and yellowish discoloration of the eyes for 3 days. She had a history of intermittent colicky upper abdominal pain once in 2 months for the last 2 years, with each episode lasting for 1–2 h, which required intravenous medication in some instances. There was no prior h/o jaundice/no similar history in other family members. She occasionally consumes beer on weekends and is a non-smoker. On examination, BMI-28 kg/m², afebrile, vital signs were stable. She was icteric, with mild tenderness in the right hypochondrium.

Lab parameters were as follows:

Parameter	Values	Parameter	Values
Hemoglobin (g/dL)	12.2	INR	1.1
Platelet count (per mm³)	220,000	Amylase (U/L)	98
Total leukocyte count (per mm³)	9600	Lipase (U/L)	121
Total bilirubin (Direct) (mg/dL)	3.2 (1.9)	S Na/K (mEq/dL)	132/4.3
AST (U/L)	115	Urea (mg/dL)	18
ALT (U/L)	122	Creatinine (mg/dL)	0.8
ALP(U/L)	450	Albumin (g/dL)	3.8

USG Abdomen: Grade II fatty liver, CBD dilated 10 mm. GB wall thickened with wall echo shadow complex.

Q. What Is the most probable diagnosis?
Ans: Choledocholithiasis.

U. V. U. Vamsidhar Reddy · A. Roy · V. Singh (✉)
Department of Hepatology, Post Graduate Institute of Medical Education and Research, Chandigarh, Punjab, India

© The Author(s), under exclusive license to Springer Nature Singapore Pte Ltd. 2022
V. Singh, A. Roy (eds.), *Clinical Rounds in Hepatology*,
https://doi.org/10.1007/978-981-16-8448-7_20

Q. What Is the sensitivity and specificity of ultrasonography and LFTs for detecting CBD stones?

Ans: USG: Sensitivity: 73%, specificity: 91% (*Gurusamy, Cochrane review, 2015*).

LFT: Bilirubin (>1.3 mg/dL) Sensitivity: 84%, specificity: 91%.

Bilirubin (>2 × ULN) Sensitivity: 42%, specificity: 97%

ALP (>125 IU/L) [Normal value: 50–170 IU/L] Sensitivity: 92%, specificity: 79%

ALP > 2 × ULN: Sensitivity: 38%, specificity: 97%

Q. What is the next best investigation to perform in this case?

Ans: EUS/MRCP

- There are no randomized trials comparing the accuracy of EUS vs. MRCP. Sensitivity (97 vs. 90%) and specificity (87 vs. 92%) for EUS and MRCP respectively (*GIE 2017*).
- The sensitivity of EUS better than MRCP for small stones, however, the specificity is similar.
- Factors impeding MRCP are claustrophobia, obesity, implanted cardiac pacemaker, or metal clips and prosthesis (ESGE 2019).
- EUS drawbacks: Risk of perforation (0.02–0.07%), prior GI bypass procedure (*ASGE 2019*).
  *ASGE: American Society for Gastrointestinal Endoscopy. *ESGE: European Society for Gastrointestinal Endoscopy

Q. When can ERCP be performed upfront in a case of Choledocholithiasis?

Ans: Patients in the ASGE *high probability group* can be subjected to an ERCP straightway.

Adapted from ASGE 2019 and ESGE 2017.

Probability	Predictors of CBD stone	Plan of action
High	USG/CT s/o choledocholithiasis or Presence of cholangitis or Serum bilirubin >4 mg/dL and dilated CBD (>6 mm with GB in situ, >8 mm post-cholecystectomy)	ERCP
Intermediate	LFT deranged Or >55 years old or USG/CT s/o dilated CBD	EUS/MRCP/intra-operative US
Low	Absence of any above-mentioned predictors	Cholecystectomy with/without intraoperative cholangioscopy or intraoperative US

Important changes in 2019 guidelines

*2010 ASGE guideline: Serum bilirubin 1.8–4.0 mg/dL and dilated CBD or bilirubin >4 mg/dL singly were considered as high-risk criteria

*Biliary pancreatitis is no longer included as an intermediate-risk criterion unlike in 2010 guidelines

Q. What are the clinical situations associated with difficult CBD stone extraction?

Ans:

Difficult CBD stones are encountered in 10–15% of ERCPs for choledocholithiasis.

   (i) Stone size > 1.5 cm, large number of stones (>10), barrel-shaped stones.
  (ii) Stones that cannot be extracted by capturing in basket or are not amenable for mechanical lithotripsy.
 (iii) Presence of complex biliary strictures, e.g., PSC, RPC.
  (iv) Hepatolithiasis, Stones in cystic duct.
   (v) Presence of surgically altered upper gut anatomy (e.g., Roux-en-Y gastric bypass and Billroth II gastro-jejunostomy).
  (vi) Presence of Mirizzi syndrome.
 (vii) Presence of periampullary diverticulum.
(viii) Shorter length of the distal CBD arm (≤36 mm), and more acute distal CBD angulation (≤135°).

High yield points:

- Laparoscopic cholecystectomy should be considered within a period of 2 weeks in patients of CBD stones, who have undergone ERCP, in order to prevent various complications viz. recurrent CBD stones, cholecystitis, biliary colic, biliary pancreatitis, and a higher risk of conversion to open cholecystectomy, which are more commonly seen in patients with a prolonged wait period.
- Antibiotic prophylaxis should be considered in the following group of patients:
  – Patients with cholangitis
  – Immune-deficient patients
  – Predicted incomplete drainage procedure
  – Patients with coexistent PSC
- Balloon catheter preferred over wire basket for stone extraction because:
  – Easy to perform
  – Occlusion cholangiography can be taken
  – No risk of entrapment in CBD
- Biliary endoprosthesis should be considered in case of
  – Partial stone clearance
  – Presence of severe acute cholangitis

- Endoscopic Papillary Balloon Dilatation preferred over endoscopic   sphincter-otomy (ES) in:
  - Presence of coagulopathy.
  - Presence of peri-ampullary diverticulum.
  - Surgically altered anatomy that increases the difficulty in the perfor-mance of ES.

Q. What are the approaches toward managing a case of large CBD Stone (>15 mm)?
Ans:

(i) Endoscopic Sphincterotomy followed by Endoscopic Papillary Balloon Dilatation.
(ii) Mechanical Lithotripsy
(iii) Intraductal Shock wave Lithotripsy
   - Electrohydraulic lithotripsy (EHL)
   - Laser lithotripsy(LL)
(iv) Extracorporeal Shock wave Lithotripsy (ESWL)

Q. What are the diagnostic criteria used for diagnosing cholangitis?
Ans: Tokyo guidelines (TG18/TG13) diagnostic criteria for acute cholangitis:

A. Presence of systemic inflammation as depicted by:
   - A-1. Presence of fever (Temperature > 38 °C) and/or shaking chills.
   - A-2. Laboratory values suggestive of inflammatory response (WBC count <4000, or >10,000; or, CRP $\geq$1 mg/dL.
B. Laboratory evidence of cholestasis
   - B-1. Jaundice (Bilirubin $\geq$2 mg/dL).
   - B-2. LFT derangement (ALP > 1.5 × ULN, GGT > 1.5 × ULN, AST > 1.5 × ULN, ALT > 1.5 × ULN).
C. Imaging
   - C-1. Dilated CBD.
   - C-2. Evidence of stricture, stone, stent, etc. on imaging.

Suspected diagnosis: 1 criterion from A + 1 criterion from either B or C.
Definite diagnosis: 1 criterion from A, 1 criterion from B, and 1 criterion from C.
Other criteria:
Charcot's triad: Right upper quadrant abdominal pain, jaundice, and fever.
Reynold's pentad: Charcot's triad with shock and altered mental status.

Q. How to assess the severity of acute cholangitis?
Ans: Severity of acute cholangitis is graded as Grade I (mild), Grade II (moderate), and Grade III (severe) according to Tokyo guidelines 2018 (TG18/13).
Grade III acute cholangitis: At least 1 of the following criteria has to be met:

1. CVS dysfunction: Defined as hypotension, with the need of vasopressors (either dopamine ≥5 µg/kg per min, or any dose of norepinephrine).
2. CNS dysfunction: Defined by altered consciousness.
3. Respiratory dysfunction: Defined as PaO2/FiO2 ratio <300.
4. Kidney dysfunction: Defined by presence of oliguria, or creatinine >2.0 mg/dL.
5. Liver dysfunction: Defined as an INR >1.5.
6. Hematological dysfunction: Defined by platelet count of <100,000/mm³.

Grade II (moderate) acute cholangitis
  Presence of at least two of the following criteria is mandatory:

1. Total leukocyte count (>12,000/mm³, or, <4000/mm³)
2. Presence of high-grade fever (defined by temperature of ≥39 °C)
3. ≥75 years old
4. Serum bilirubin ≥5 mg/dL
5. Serum albumin <0.73 × ULN

  Grade I (mild) acute cholangitis
  Patients with cholangitis who does not fulfill the criteria for Grade II or III cholangitis are said to have Grade I (mild) acute cholangitis.

Q. How to Manage a Case of Choledocholithiasis with Cholangitis?
Ans:

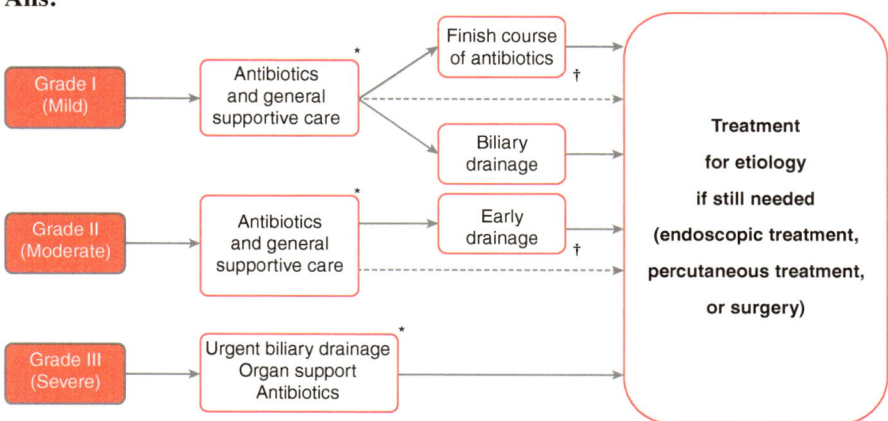

Adapted from ASGE guidelines
*Blood culture should be sent before starting antibiotics.
  During biliary drainage, bile samples should be taken and sent for culture and sensitivity testing.
  †**Principles of treatment for acute cholangitis:**

- Antibiotics
- Biliary drainage
- Treatment of the underlying cause

Patients with CBD stones presenting as mild or moderate cholangitis, CBD clearance should be considered during initial biliary drainage procedure, if possible.

Q. Which antibiotics are commonly used to treat biliary infection? Which antibiotics have good biliary penetration?

Good penetration efficiency (ABSCR > 1)	Low penetration efficiency (ABSCR < 1)
Piperacillin/Tazobactum (4.8)	Ceftriaxone (0.75)
Tigecycline (>10)	Cefotaxime (0.23)
Amoxicillin/clavulanate (1.1)	Meropenem (0.38)
Ciprofloxacin (>5)	Ceftazidime (0.18)
Ampicillin/sulbactam (2.4)	Vancomycin (0.41)
Cefepime (2.04)	Amikacin (0.54)
Levofloxacin (1.6)	Gentamicin (0.3)
Penicillin G (>5)	
Imipenem (1.01)	

ABSCR Antibiotics Bile/Serum Concentration Ratio

Further Reading

Manes G, et al. Endoscopic management of common bile duct stones: European Society of Gastrointestinal Endoscopy (ESGE) guideline. Endoscopy. 2019;51(05):472–91.

Dumonceau JM, et al. Endoscopic biliary stenting: indications, choice of stents, and results: European Society of Gastrointestinal Endoscopy (ESGE) Clinical Guideline—Updated October 2017. Endoscopy. 2018;50(9):910–30.

Prasanta Debnath, Akash Roy, and Virendra Singh

A previously healthy 39-year-old female patient presented with right-sided abdominal pain and jaundice with associated pruritus, clay-colored stools, and fatigue for 14 days. No history of fever, anorexia, weight loss, nausea, vomiting. She had history of cholecystectomy 1 year back. She denied any previous episodes of jaundice or weight loss. On admission, physical examination revealed scleral icterus. She was afebrile. The abdomen was soft, non-tender, and liver and spleen were not palpable.

Investigations

Parameter	Values	Parameter	Values
Hemoglobin	11.2	INR	1.4
Platelet count	298	HBsAg	NR
Total leukocyte count	7000	Anti-HCV	NR
Total bilirubin (Direct)	10.8 (7.0)	AMA/pANCA	Neg
AST	98	S Na/K	137/4.3
ALT	48	Urea	32
ALP	566	Creatinine	0.8
Albumin	3.9	CA 19-9	12

USG Abdomen: Liver 16 cm, enlarged, bilateral central and peripheral IHBRD, dilated CHD with distal CBD being normal. Pancreas and spleen: normal.

P. Debnath
Department of Gastroenterology, TNMC and BYL Nair Charitable Hospital, Mumbai, India

A. Roy · V. Singh (✉)
Department of Hepatology, Post Graduate Institute of Medical Education and Research, Chandigarh, Punjab, India

Q. What Is the most probable diagnosis based on the given vignette?
Ans: Extrahepatic obstructive jaundice due to post-cholecystectomy biliary stricture.

Q. How do you differentiate between benign and malignant biliary stricture clinically?
Ans:
Benign vs. Malignant:
Clinical and laboratory clues:

Favors benign etiology	Favors malignant etiology
Young patient without any weight loss	Unintentional weight loss + Poor general well being
Cholangitis more frequent	Cholangitis less frequent H/O PSC (primary sclerosing cholangitis) or decompensation in known PSC patient
H/O gall stone disease	Long stricture >1 cm
Higher IgG4 level (In suspected Immunoglobulin G4 disease)	Asymmetrical stricture
? Normal CA 19-9	? Raised CA 19-9
H/O cholecystectomy or hepatobiliary surgery	Presence of anomalous pancreatobiliary junction
H/O Trauma	H/O choledochal cyst
Stable weight	Short course without antecedent illness
Fluctuation in laboratory parameters	Progressive disease without fluctuation

Additional points:

- In postoperative setting (cholecystectomy/hepatobiliary surgery), an acute presentation indicates iatrogenic bile duct injury/biliary stricture.
- Presentation during an episode of acute pancreatitis may indicate stone-related biliary obstruction.
- A gradual presentation evolving in <3 months generally indicates an inflammatory process, which is likely to improve in due course.
- However, symptom duration >3 months after an insult/injury generally indicates a more fibrotic stricture, which is less likely to improve with time and may require more aggressive therapy (endoscopic/surgical).
- Malignancy should be suspected when there is an occult/delayed presentation and no risk factors are identified.
- Waxing waning clinical picture or laboratory abnormalities generally suggest a benign stricture, whereas a progressive disease course is indicative of an underlying malignant etiology.

Laboratory features:

- Elevated ALP (alkaline phosphatase) with normal transaminase or serum bilirubin is suggestive of intra- or extrahepatic bile duct obstruction.
- Elevated aminotransferases with ALP and/or bilirubin indicate simultaneous presence of hepatitis, or an acute presentation of CBD obstruction.
- Complete CBD obstruction + healthy liver, i.e., without any hepatocellular injury, serum bilirubin usually remains below 20 mg/dL.
- Bilirubin >20 mg/dL indicates associated hepatocellular injury, in the presence/absence of biliary obstruction.
- Long-standing obstruction with jaundice may lead to fat maldigestion and malabsorption, as well as deficiency of fat-soluble vitamins, including vitamin K, leading to elevated PT/INR.

Q. What are the cholangiographic features of malignancy?
Cholangiographic features of malignancy:

1. Progressive focal stricturing over time
2. Abrupt shelf-like borders
3. Length of stricture >14 mm
4. Presence of IHBR (intrahepatic biliary radicle) dilation
5. Intraductal polypoid or nodular mass on cholangiogram

In the setting of PSC with dominant stricture:

1. Length of stricture >1 cm
2. Location: at bifurcation of CHD
3. Irregular margins on cholangiogram

Q. What are the common causes of Benign Biliary Stricture? (Table 21.1)

Table 21.1 Differential diagnosis of benign biliary stricture

Common	Less common
Primary sclerosing cholangitis	Bile-duct ischemia
Chronic pancreatitis	Vasculitis: SLE- and ANCA-associated
Post-cholecystectomy stricture	Radiation therapy
Bilioenteric anastomosis	Portal cavernoma cholangiopathy
Inflammatory strictures	Tuberculosis
IgG4 cholangiopathy	Post-sphincterotomy
Post-liver transplantation	Trauma
	Mirizzi syndrome
	Parasitic infection
	AIDS cholangiopathy
	Post-radiofrequency ablation

Table 21.2 Points of differentiation of intra- and extrahepatic cholestasis

Points	Intra-hepatic	Extra-hepatic
Pruritus	More severe	Less severe
Cholangitis	−	+
Pain abdomen	+	++
Decompensated liver disease	++	+ (in cases with secondary biliary cirrhosis)
H/O surgery/endoscopic intervention	−	++
H/O recent CAM/antibiotic use	+/−	−
Prodrome with anorexia, nausea, vomiting	+/−	−
H/O travel, sexual contact, blood transfusion, or intravenous drug use	+/−	−
Presence of an abdominal lump	−	+

Q. How do you differentiate between the Intra- and Extrahepatic Causes for Cholestasis? (Table 21.2)

Q. State Courvoisiers Law

Ans: Ludwig Courvoisier stated, "with obstruction of the common duct by a stone, dilatation is rare. The organ is usually well shrunken. With obstruction from other kinds, on the contrary, distension is the rule. Shrinking occurs in only one-twelfth of cases."

No mention of malignancy, nor regarding the site of the biliary obstruction was made in the original statement.

Q. Mention the Exceptions to Courvoisiers Law

- Double impaction of calculi, one obstructing the cystic duct and the other occluding the distal CBD. The CBD stone causes biliary obstruction and a stone in the cystic duct leads to mucocele or empyema of gall bladder, leading to palpable GB.
- Pancreatic stone obstructing the ampulla.
- Recurrent pyogenic cholangitis.
- Periampullary malignancy in post-cholecystectomy patient.
- Mirizzi syndrome.

Q. How to investigate a case of indeterminate biliary stricture?

Ans: Indeterminate biliary stricture is defined as biliary stricture, which remains undiagnosed when basic workup including transabdominal imaging (USG/CT/MRI) and ERCP with routine cytological brushing are non-diagnostic.

- Incidence: 20% of biliary strictures are labelled as indeterminate.
- 25% of stricture operated as malignant turns out to be benign.

Diagnosis:
Tools for investigation
ERCP

- Tissue sampling (Brush cytology)
- Intraductal forceps biopsy
- Intraductal transmucosal (trans-papillary) ERCP-FNA
- Cholangioscopy with forceps biopsy

EUS: FNA, IDUS
CT
MRI
PET scan
Brush cytology: Overall brush cytology are cheap and readily available but given the potential pauci-cellular nature of tumors and difficulties in tissue targeting and acquisition are overall poorly sensitive. Shown to have a sensitivity of 30–60% and specificity of 60–90%. Results are usually classified as positive, negative, or suggestive of atypical cells. Atypical cells are common result in biliary brush cytology, especially in primary sclerosing cholangitis and may lead to need for resampling.
Bonus point:
ABBS Score (Atypical Biliary Brushing Score): Score ≥4 associated with malignancy (Witt et al., Diag Cyto, 2012).

Variables	Score
Age ≥ 60	+1
Endoscopic impression malignant	+2
Procedure indication: pancreatic mass	+1
Stricture in CHD	+2
Stricture in distal CBD	+1
Presence of PSC	+2
CA-19-9 >300 U/mL	+1

Both brush cytology and intraductal biopsy have comparable diagnostic specificity with limited sensitivity (Sensitivity 45% and 48%, respectively). The combination of both lead to modest increase in sensitivity (59%) (Navaneethan et al., GIE, 2015).

Q. Mention novel sampling and processing techniques in the evaluation of Indeterminate Biliary Stricture

Smash protocol: Crushing of serial forceps biopsy samples between slides followed by fixation, staining (Papanicolaou), and on-site evaluation. Sensitivity 76%, specificity 100% (Wright AJG, 2011).

Advanced analytical methods:

(a) Fluorescent In-situ Hybridization (FISH)
(b) Digital Image Analysis
(c) Flow cytometry
(d) Next Generation Sequencing (genomic alterations—KRAS, TP53, CDKN2A, SMAD) 4) Biliseq (28 genes)
(e) Extracellular vesicles

FISH:

- Detect polysomic cells before other tests.
- Meta-analysis: FISH in PSC sensitivity: 68%, specificity: 70% (Navaneethan et al., GIE, 2014)
- Combined triple assessment (standard brush cytology, intraductal biopsy, FISH): sensitivity: 82%, specificity 100%. (Nanda et al., Ther Adv Gastro, 2015)

Q. What are the Advanced Imaging Tools for the Evaluation of Indeterminate Biliary Stricture?

1. **EUS**

   Features suggestive of malignancy:

   - Presence of hypoechoic mass.
   - Bile duct wall thickness > 3 mm.
     Sensitivity 79%; specificity: 79%; PPV: 73%; NPV: 80% (Lee et al., AJG, 2004).
   - EUS better than triphasic CT and MRI for tumor detection.
   - EUS identifies 100% of distal & 83% hilar tumors (Mohamadnejad et al., GIE, 2011).
   - EUS FNA for diagnosis of CCA: sensitivity 73% (distal better than hilar; 81% vs. 59%).
   - With percutaneous as well as EUS guided FNA the risk of tumor seeding of needle track increases, thus making potentially transplant ineligible.

2. **Intra-ductal Ultrasound (IDUS)**

Features suggestive of benign disease	Features suggestive of malignancy
Hyperechoic lesion	Hypoechoic mass, irregular margin
Symmetric wall thickening	Asymmetric (eccentric) wall thickening
Sharp demarcation with surrounding tissues	Poorly demarcated borders
Preserved tissue planes	Abrupt shoulders
Smooth edges	Disruption of normal triple-layer architecture
	Invasion of adjacent structures
	Papillary surface
	Malignant appearing peri-ductal lymph nodes

3. **Cholangioscopy**

Indications in biliary stricture:

- Discrimination of indeterminate biliary lesions
- Tissue acquisition under direct visual control
- Delineation of intraductal tumor margin of CCA
- Targeted cannulation of complex strictures
- Therapeutic applications

Clues for biliary malignancy on cholangioscopy:

- Dilated and tortuous mucosal vessels.
- Intraductal nodular or papillary lesions.
- Oozing and irregular surface.
- Vascular pattern-"Tumor vessel" sign for malignancy is highly specific in patients with indeterminate stricture.

Cholangioscopic findings in various biliary tract lesions:

Lesions	Cholangioscopic findings
Normal	Flat surface Pseudo-diverticula ± Normal vessels (Regular network)
Inflammatory	Bumpy surface Pseudo-diverticulae + Intra diverticular calculi ± Regular granular lesions (hyperplasia) Tortuous vessels (dilated/non-dilated) without encasement or fusion of vessels Scarring
Neoplasms	Irregular papillary or granular lesions Nodular lesions Friable mucosa with easy bleeding Tortuous vessels (dilated/non-dilated) with fusion/encasement

4. Confocal laser endomicroscopy (CLE)

Probe-based CLE (pCLE) via ERCP: Sensitivity 89%, specificity 71%.
Paris criteria:

Normal bile duct	1. Reticular network of thin dark branching bands (<20 micron)—thin collagen bundle 2. Light gray background—lymphatic sinuses 3. Vessels (<20 micron)
Inflammatory stricture	1. Multiple white bands—vessels 2. Dark granular pattern in scales 3. Enlarged space between scales 4. Thickened reticular structures
Malignant stricture	1. Thick white bands (>20 micron)—vessels 2. Thick dark bands (>40 micron) 3. Epithelium 4. Dark clumps

Further Reading

Bowlus CL, et al. Evaluation of indeterminate biliary strictures. Nat Rev Gastroenterol Hepatol. 2016;13(1):28.

Prasanta Debnath, Akash Roy, and Virendra Singh

Case Vignette A 42-year-old woman presents to the emergency department with worsening epigastric pain, nausea, vomiting of 12-h duration. The pain is sharp, severe, and radiates to the back. History of intermittent RUQ pain lasting for 2–3 h since last year which used to get relieved with NSAID. She is non-addict, known hypertensive on tablet Amlodipine for 3 years. On examination, her BMI is 27 kg/m^2, she is afebrile, BP-98/60; PR 110/min; abdomen is distended, and is tympanic to percussion. There is tenderness to deep palpation in the epigastrium. There is no lump or organomegaly. There is no presence of any free fluid.

Investigations

Parameter	Values	Parameter	Values
Hemoglobin	11.8	INR	1.1
Hematocrit	38%	CRP	25
Platelet count	354	Amylase	780
Total leukocyte count	12,000	Lipase	1200
Total bilirubin (Direct)	1.2 (0.6)	Calcium	9.2
AST	102	S Na/K	132/4.3
ALT	152	BUN	28
ALP	348	Creatinine	1
Albumin	3.8		

P. Debnath
Department of Gastroenterology, TNMC and BYL Nair Charitable Hospital, Mumbai, India

A. Roy · V. Singh (✉)
Department of Hepatology, Post Graduate Institute of Medical Education and Research, Chandigarh, Punjab, India

© The Author(s), under exclusive license to Springer Nature Singapore Pte Ltd. 2022
V. Singh, A. Roy (eds.), *Clinical Rounds in Hepatology*,
https://doi.org/10.1007/978-981-16-8448-7_22

USG abdomen: Multiple GB calculi, CBD 6 mm, pancreas—bulky head with peripancreatic edema and mild ascites. Liver: Normal. No IHBRD.

Q.What Is the most likely diagnosis?
Ans: Acute Gall stone-induced Pancreatitis.

Q. What are the markers of severe disease in case of Acute Pancreatitis (AP)?
Ans:
Patient-related factors:

- Age > 55 years
- High BMI
- Presence of other comorbidities

Clinical characteristics

- Painless presentation (5–10%)
- Presence of Grey-Turner's sign and Cullen's sign (<1%)
- Altered sensorium
- Presence of Systemic Inflammatory Response Syndrome (SIRS): 2 of following:
  - PR > 90/min
  - RR > 20/min (PaCO2 < 32 mm Hg)
  - Temperature > 38/<36 °C
  - WBC count > 12,000/<4000 or band forms >10%
- Reduced urine output
- Presence of breathing difficulty
- Presence of ascites

Laboratory features:

- Increasing BUN (blood urea nitrogen) level or BUN > 20 mg/dl
- Serum creatinine > ULN (upper limit of normal)
- Rising hematocrit or absolute value > 44%
- Raised lipase (7 × ULN) in pediatric AP
- D-dimer in pediatric AP
- CRP > 15 mg/dl
- Phospholipase A2 (degrades pulmonary surfactant, may play role in respiratory dysfunction in AP)
- Procalcitonin
- Miscellaneous—TNF-α, Thrombopoietin, Carboxypeptidase-B activation peptide, PMN elastase, Hepcidin, etc.

Imaging Findings:

- Presence of pleural effusion(s)

- Presence of pulmonary infiltrate(s)
- Presence of extrapancreatic fluid collections (multiple/extensive)
- Various EUS features such as:
  - Diffuse pancreatic parenchymal edema
  - Peri-parenchymal plastering
  - Diffuse retroperitoneal free fluid, and peri-pancreatic edema

Q. How is the diagnosis of acute pancreatitis made?
Ans:
   According to the Revised Atlanta Criteria of 2012 (updated from 1992): two of the following three criteria are needed for a diagnosis of acute pancreatitis:

1. Pain abdomen consistent with acute pancreatitis
2. Pancreatic enzymes—lipase or amylase $\geq 3 \times$ ULN
3. Characteristic features of acute pancreatitis on imaging—USG or cross-sectional imaging CT, or MRI.

Q. What are the features of abdominal pain in AP?
Ans:
   Pain abdomen:

- **Site:** Pain usually involves the entire upper abdomen. Lower abdominal pain may result from spread of pancreatic exudation along left colon.
- **Onset:** Rapid, with maximal intensity reached within 10–20 min.
- **Characteristics:** Steady and moderate to very severe, unbearable, and boring.
- **Radiation:** Band-like radiation of the pain to the back occurs in around 50% of the cases.
- **Associated features:** Nausea and vomiting in 90%.

Q. What are the physical examination findings in AP?
General physical examination:

- Evidence of SIRS (systemic inflammatory response syndrome)
- BP: Initially higher than normal then hypotension due to third space loss and hypovolemia.
- Temperature: Initially normal, may rise to 101–103 °F (1–3 days) with onset of SIRS.
- Tachypnea with shallow respiration (due to subdiaphragmatic exudate).
- Dyspnea due to pulmonary causes like pleural effusions, atelectasis, ARDS, or cardiac cause—heart failure.

- Icterus: CBD calculi (gall stone pancreatitis) or distal CBD obstruction from edematous pancreatic head, or compression by pseudocyst, or from coexistent liver disease.
- Uncommon clinical findings in AP include subcutaneous nodular fat necrosis along with polyarthritis (PPP syndrome-Panniculitis Polyarthritis, Pancreatitis syndrome).
- Purtscher retinopathy: Patient complains of visual abnormalities, including blindness. Pathogenesis: microembolization in the retinal vessels. Fundus examination reveals cotton wool spots, retinal hemorrhages, and edema, located around the optic disc.

Systemic examination:
In mild pancreatitis:

- Mild abdominal tenderness.
- Guarding usually absent.
  In severe pancreatitis:

- Tender abdomen
- Abdominal distension (due to ileus), located mainly in the upper abdomen.
- Guarding: usually present and marked in the upper part.
- Rigidity can be present.
- Bowel sounds: Reduced/ absent (due to ileus).

Additional abdominal findings may include:

- Cullen's sign: Superficial edema and bruising in the subcutaneous fatty tissue around the umbilicus.
- Grey Turner's sign: Bluish/ecchymotic discoloration of the lateral abdominal wall or flanks. Usually occurs 24–48 h after the onset of acute pancreatitis.
- Both Cullen's and Grey Turner's signs are due to extravasation of hemorrhagic exudate to the respective areas.
- Palpable abdominal mass from pseudocyst or large inflammatory peri-pancreatic fluid collection.

Physical findings that point to a specific cause of AP:

- Hepatomegaly, spider angiomas, and Dupuytren's contracture and other stigmata of chronic liver disease favor alcoholic pancreatitis.
- Xanthomas, xanthelasma, and lipemia retinalis usually suggest hyperlipidemic pancreatitis.
- Parotid pain and swelling in mumps.
- Band keratopathy (an infiltration on the lateral margin of the cornea) can be seen in patients with hypercalcemia.

Q. What are the clinical scores to assess severity of this patient?
Ans:

1. **Revised Atlanta Classification**

	Mild	Moderately severe	Severe
Organ failure	No	Resolving < 48 h	Persistent > 48 h
Local/systemic complications	No	Without persistent organ failure	Single/Multiple organ failure
Mortality	0.1%	2.1%	52.2%

Local complications: Peri-pancreatic fluid collections, peri-pancreatic necrosis, pancreatic necrosis (sterile/infected), pseudocyst, WON (walled off necrosis) (sterile/infected).
Organ failure: Defined by modified Marshall Scoring System:

Organ system	0	1	2	3	4
Respiratory (PaO2/FiO2)	>400	301–400	201–300	101–200	<101
Renal (Creatinine) mg/dl	<1.4	1.4–1.8	1.9–3.6	3.6–4.9	>4.9
Cardiovascular Systolic BP (mm Hg)	>90	<90; fluid responsive	<90; not fluid responsive	<90 pH<7.3	<90 pH<7.2

Organ failure is defined as a score of ≥2 for one of these organ systems.

2. **Determinant-Based Classification**

Based on organ failure (defined by SOFA score ≥ 2) and status of peri-pancreatic necrosis.

	Mild	Moderate	Severe	Critical
Peri-pancreatic necrosis	No and	Sterile and/or	Infected or	Infected and
Organ failure	No	Transient	Persistent	Persistent
Mortality	0.1%	4%	39.2%	54.1%

3. **BISAP Score:** Bedside Index of Severity of Acute Pancreatitis; 5 parameters-1 point for each component.
   (a) **BUN > 25 mg/dl**
   (b) **Impaired mental status**
   (c) **SIRS**
   (d) **Age > 60 years**
   (e) **Pleural effusion**
        Score 0 and 5, mortality <1% and 22%, respectively.
4. **Ranson Criteria:** Score > 3, mortality 62%

5. **APACHE II Score**
6. **Glasgow Imrie Score**
7. **PANC-3 Score**

CT Severity Scores

1. CT Severity Index

Balthazar grades	Definition	Points
A	Normal pancreas	0
B	Focal or diffuse enlargement + contour irregularities and inhomogeneous attenuation	1
C	Grade B + peripancreatic inflammation	2
D	Grade C + single fluid collection	3
E	Grade C plus ≥2 peripancreatic fluid collections or gas in the pancreas or retroperitoneum	4
CTSI=Balthazar Grade Points Plus Necrosis Score		
Necrosis score	**Points**	
No necrosis	0	
Necrosis <33% pancreatic parenchyma	2	
Necrosis 33–50%	4	
Necrosis of >50%	6	

Highest possible score: 4 (Balthazar grade E) + 6 (necrosis of >50%) = 10 points

Score 0–6, mortality 3.8%; score>6, mortality 18%

2. Modified CT Severity Index

CT Grade	Points	Necrosis	Points	Extra-pancreatic complications	Points
Normal parenchyma	0	0	0	Ascites	2
Intrinsic parenchymal abnormality ±peripancreatic inflammation	2	≤30%	2	Pleural effusion Vascular complications GIT involvement Extra-pancreatic parenchymal abnormalities	
Pancreatic/peri-pancreatic fluid collection or peri-pancreatic fat necrosis	4	>30%	4		

Modified Severity Index= CT Grade+percentage necrosis+extra-pancreatic complications:
Mild (0–2)
Moderate (4–6)
Severe (8–10)

3. **Extra-pancreatic Inflammation on CT (EPIC) Score**
   Pleural effusion
   (a) None: 0
   (b) Unilateral: 1
   (c) Bilateral: 2
   Ascites
   (a) None: 0
   (b) Unilateral: 1
   (c) Bilateral: 2
   Retro-peritoneal inflammation:
   (a) None: 0
   (b) Unilateral: 1
   (c) Bilateral: 2
   Mesenteric inflammation:
   (a) None: 0
   (b) Present: 1
   Score ≥ 3, Severe Pancreatitis

Q. How to differentiate between alcohol associated AP from gall stone Pancreatitis?
Ans:

	Alcoholic AP	Gall stone Pancreatitis
Demographics	Male Age 40 years 5–10 years heavy alcohol consumption	Female Age > 40 years
Recurrent attacks	More common	30–50% without cholecystectomy (average time 108 days)
Lab test	AST > ALT High MCV	ALT > 150 (3 × ULN)- 96% specificity, sensitivity 48%

Q. What is the most common systemic complication associated with AP?
Ans: Respiratory insufficiency.

Q. What are the pathogenetic mechanisms of hypocalcemia in acute pancreatitis?
Ans: Low serum albumin (the most important cause)
   Hypomagnesemia
   Calcium-soap formation
   Endocrine disturbance involving parathyroid hormone, calcitonin, and glucagon
   Calcium binding by free fatty acid–albumin complexes
   Intracellular calcium migration
   Endotoxinemia.

Q. What are the management options for this patient?

Ans: Management of AP according to time frame:

- First 72 h
- 4–7 days
- 2nd–3rd week
- >4th week

Early treatment:

A. Fluid resuscitation.
B. Pain control.
A. Initially, patients may appear clinically well. However, they can deteriorate rapidly if window of opportunity for resuscitation is missed (first 24 h).

Fluid loss in AP:
At 48 h (Ranson et al., 1974):

- Mild: 3.7 l
- Severe: 5.6 l

Median fluid loss in AP: 3.2 l

Recommended fluid administration in AP: 15–20 ml/kg bolus followed by 1.5–3 ml/kg/h, depending on response.

Which fluid is to be chosen?

NS (normal saline) could lead to a large chloride load contributing to kidney injury. Hyperchloremic metabolic acidosis due to NS (pH 5.5) could promote inflammation. Lactate has been found to downregulate inflammatory cascade by negatively regulating TLR induction of the NLRP3 inflammasome pathway and production of IL1β. Calcium in Ringer's lactate could reduce early systemic inflammation by binding non-esterified fatty acids.

Aims of fluid therapy:

- Mean arterial pressure (MAP): 70 mm Hg
- Hematocrit (Hct) 40–42%
- Urine output (UO) 0.5–1 ml/min

A goal-directed strategy using clinical parameters (MAP, pulse rate, UO) rather than specific lab parameters (Hct, BUN) is recommended.

B. **Pain control:**

- Adequate analgesia is very important.
- Uncontrolled pain has a negative effect on microvasculature (Induction of vasoconstriction).
- Opioids (Pentazocine) are better than NSAIDs (Garg et al., AJG, 2019).

C. **Nutrition:**

Enteral feeding should be primary therapy in patients with predicted severe AP. Types of feed:

- Oral/enteral (NG/NJ)
- 25–30 kcal/kg with 1.2–2 g protein/kg
- Rarely TPN

AGA recommends early feeding (usually within 24 h) for all patients with AP (mild, moderately severe, and severe) as per patient tolerance.

RCTs have shown similar outcomes if feeding is initiated within 24 h vs. 72 h (Backer et al., NEJM, 2014).

Enteral feeding is better than parenteral, because

- Less complications
- Less requirement of surgery
- Reduced mortality
- Maintains the structural and functional integrity of GIT

NG feeding is similar to NJ feeding (Meta-analysis Chang et al., Critical Care, 2013).

However, NJ's theoretical advantage is that it provides more rest to the pancreas via the ileal brake mechanism. NG is easier, but many patients don't tolerate NG feeding.

NJ is indicated in:

- Critically ill patients with increased risk of aspiration pneumonia
- Gastroparesis
- Intolerant to NG feeding

D. **Prophylactic antibiotics**:

Meta-analysis showed no benefit (Jiang et al., WJG, 2012).

Most patients in India get prophylactic antibiotics (66%) (Talukdar et al., IJG, 2014).

Prophylactic antibiotics associated with:

- More resistant infections
- Gram-positive infections
- More fungal infections

E. Miscellaneous

- Respiratory care
- Cardiovascular care
- Management of metabolic complications (Hyperglycemia, hypocalcemia, hypomagnesemia)

Diagnosis of (Peri)-Pancreatic Collections and Infected Necrosis:
Pancreatic necrosis

Definition: Lack of enhancement of pancreatic parenchyma on CECT.

Incidence: 5–10% of AP episodes.

Location: Pancreas alone, extrapancreatic tissues alone, or both (most common).

Diagnosis: Presence or absence of pancreatic necrosis is best diagnosed by CECT after 72 h of presentation.

Local complications of AP have been defined in the revised Atlanta classification There are four types of collections associated with AP.

	Interstitial edematous pancreatitis	Necrotizing pancreatitis
<4 weeks	**Acute (peri)pancreatic fluid collection:** Homogenous fluid adjacent to pancreas without a recognizable wall.	**Acute necrotic collection:** Intra- and/or extra-pancreatic necrotic collection without a well-defined wall.
>4 weeks	**Pancreatic pseudocyst** An encapsulated well-defined, usually extra-pancreatic fluid collection with minimal solids.	**Walled-off necrosis** Intra- and/or extra-pancreatic necrotic collection with a well-defined wall.

Q. What are the indications for intervention in necrotizing pancreatitis?
Ans:

Indications for Intervention in Necrotizing Pancreatitis (Radiological, Endoscopic, or Surgical):

1. Infected necrotizing pancreatitis (either documented on culture or clinical suspicion) with clinical worsening, preferably after 4 weeks after the necrotic collection has been well encapsulated.
2. Persistent organ failure for several weeks.
3. Non-infected WON with any one of the following indications:
    (a) Gastric outlet obstruction, intestinal obstruction, or CBD obstruction.
    (b) Ongoing symptoms (e.g., pain abdomen, "persistent unwellness") continued systemic illness, loss of appetite, loss of weight.
    (c) Completely disrupted pancreatic duct with ongoing symptoms.

Rare indications for interventions include:

- Abdominal compartment syndrome
- Gastrointestinal bleeding
- Bowel ischemia

Asymptomatic WON does not warrant any intervention regardless of the size and extension of the collection as they may spontaneously resolve over time.

Q. Why Is It advisable to intervene after 4 Weeks after onset of symptoms in case of WON?
Ans:

(a) Allow liquefaction: Predominant solid necrotic component is found initially, which are poorly demarcated from surrounding viable tissue.
(b) Allow encapsulation: Collection at this stage is not encapsulated. Hence, it is associated with more complications like pneumoperitoneum, pneumo-retroperitoneum, and more infective complications.

Q. Indications for emergent intervention
Abdominal compartment syndrome: Life-saving radiological or surgical decompression should be considered once medical management fails.
   Other indications for emergency surgery include:

• Hollow viscus perforation
• Severe bleeding refractory to medial, endoscopic, or radiologic (angiographic) intervention
• Bowel infarction

Q. What are the various strategies for intervention in pancreatic necrotic collection?
Ans: Minimally invasive endoscopic and surgical step-up techniques have replaced aggressive treatment modalities like open surgical debridement, which used to be traditionally employed for infected pancreatic necrosis in the past. Risk of acute complications like peri-operative stress, organ failure, and chronic ones like external pancreatic fistulae, pancreatic exocrine and endocrine deficiency, and hernias (incisional) are less commonly seen with newer modalities.
   Minimally invasive necrosectomy classification:

A. **Method of visualization**
     1. Open
     2. Radiologic
     3. Endoscopic
     4. Hybrid, or other
B. **Route**
     1. Peroral
         (a) Transpapillary
         (b) Transmural
     2. Percutaneous retroperitoneal
     3. Percutaneous transperitoneal, with or without transmural puncture
 First-line treatment for infected necrosis:

Current standard of care for infected necrotizing pancreatitis: Step-up approach of PCD f/b on-demand necrosectomy in the later phase of illness when the necrotic collection becomes organized (Based on TENSION trial, Brunschot et al., The Lancet, 2018).

Endoscopic transluminal drainage (ETD) or image-guided percutaneous catheter drainage, preferably via a retroperitoneal approach, followed by endoscopic or minimally invasive surgical necrosectomy as needed (IAP/APA guidelines, Pancreatology, 2013).

Summary of Randomized Controlled Trials Comparing Endoscopic and Minimally Invasive Surgical Step-Up Approach:

	PENGUIN trial		TENSION trial		MISER trial	
Modality	Endoscopic	Surgical	Endoscopic	Surgical	Endoscopic	Surgical
Patients, *n*	10	10	51	47	34	32
Infected necrosis (%)	100	90	45	57	91	94
Death %	10	40	18	13	9	6
End-point %	20	80	43	45	12	41
Complications						
Bleeding (%)	0	0	22	21	0	9
Perforation (%)	0	20	8	17	0	0
Fistula (%)	10	70	5	32	0	28

Q. What are the various complications of severe AP?

A. **Pancreatic fistulae**.

External pancreatic fistulae: Persistent fluid drainage via percutaneous drain (PCD), PCD tract, or surgical wound site, with amylase > 3× serum value. Pancreatic fistula usually closes after 10 weeks (median duration).

Management:

Transpapillary stent to bridge the site of leakage [effective in 27% (9–69%)] (Arvanitakis et al., Endoscopy, 2008). Transpapillary stents may diminish the chances of recurrent fluid collection after resolution.

Endoscopic transpapillary stenting vs. conservative management: Rates of fistula closure same (84 vs. 75 %) but a shorter median time to resolve (71 vs. 120 days) (Bakker et al., Ann Surg, 2011).

B. **Disconnected Pancreatic Duct Syndrome (DPDS)**

Important complication of acute necrotizing pancreatitis (ANP).

Forms as a result of necrosis of the MPD, resulting in discontinuation between viable upstream pancreatic parenchyma and duodenum.

Incidence of DPDS: 16–46.3%

Most common site: Neck of the pancreas
The diagnostic criteria of DPDS (Rana S, Pancreatology, 2020):

- Necrosis of at least 2 cm of the pancreas (<2 cm is usually associated with the development of stricture of PD and not complete disconnection).
- Pancreatic parenchyma distal to the site of necrosis must be viable.
- Free extravasation of contrast agent (dye) on pancreatogram during ERCP with total cut-off of the MPD.

Complications of DPDS:

1. Recurrent fluid collection
Acute and chronic pancreatitis of the distal pancreatic parenchyma: Occurs long term after resolution of necrotizing pancreatitis. It results due to scarring of the upstream duct with resultant closed-space obstruction and complications.
2. Diabetes mellitus (More with proximal—head/genu DPD compared to body/tail).

Management:

1. Long-standing indwelling DPSs placed during transmural drainage.
2. Prophylactic trans-papillary PD stenting during transluminal drainage and/or necrosectomy.
3. For chronic DPDS:
   (a) Surgical resection of the upstream gland with or without islet cell autotransplantation to reduce risk of diabetes.
   (b) Roux-en-Y PJ: If the upstream PD is amenable for PJ.
   (c) EUS-guided pancreaticogastrostomy.

C. **Exocrine and endocrine insufficiency:**
Acute necrotizing pancreatitis is commonly associated with exocrine pancreatic insufficiency. Pooled prevalence: 27.1% at 36 months (Hollemans et al., Pancreatology, 2018). Pancreatic enzyme replacement therapy may be beneficial during the early refeeding phase.
Endocrine insufficiency:
Pooled prevalence of prediabetes, diabetes mellitus (DM), and insulin requirement after acute pancreatitis: 16%, 23%, and 15%, respectively (Das et al., Gut, 2014).
The mechanism of endocrine insufficiency is unrelated to the severity of pancreatitis, reflecting pathophysiologic pathways other than necrosis.

D. **Splanchnic vein thrombosis (SVT)**

Incidence: 16–18% of cases with necrotizing pancreatitis.
Location: splenic vein (most common), portal vein, superior mesenteric vein.

Clinical features:

- Mainly asymptomatic (with isolated splenic vein involvement)
- Torrential upper GI variceal bleeding
- Ascites

Management: Symptomatic treatment of complications to be considered.

Role of anticoagulation: Controversial data exist in literature. Recanalization rate not statistically significant in patients treated with anticoagulants. Not recommended in patients with isolated splenic vein involvement.

E. **Pseudoaneurysm**.

Arterial pseudoaneurysm results from erosion of walls of surrounding arteries by necrotic collection. Direct injury to adjacent vessels can also be caused by percutaneous drains, LAMS, and during endoscopic or surgical necrosectomy.

Peripancreatic pseudoaneurysm classification:

Type of artery	Communication with GIT	Exposure to pancreatic juice
I. Minor artery >5 mm away from a major artery	A. No communication	1. No exposure
II. Major artery which may be sacrificed	B. Communication +	2. Exposure +
III. Major artery which cannot be sacrificed		

Most common location of pseudoaneurysms:

- Splenic artery (most common) (35–50%)
- Gastroduodenal
- Pancreaticoduodenal (20–25%).

Risk of rupture of pseudoaneurysm is much higher compared to aneurysm of comparable size due to poor support of the aneurysm wall, and are associated with significant morbidity and mortality.

Management:

Trans-arterial embolization ± pseudoaneurysm stenting. Cyanoacrylate glue, ethiodized oil, gel foam, thrombin, polyvinyl alcohol injection, or coil can also be placed for better hemostasis.

Further Reading

Dijk V, et al. Acute pancreatitis: recent advances through randomised trials. Gut. 2017;66(11):2024–32.

Crockett SD, et al. American Gastroenterological Association Institute guideline on initial management of acute pancreatitis. Gastroenterology. 2018;154(4):1096–101.

Chronic Pancreatitis

Babu Lal Meena, Akash Roy, and Virendra Singh

Q. What are the commonly used definitions for Chronic Pancreatitis (CP)?
The classical definition of CP was the "Cambridge definition" (1984) which defined CP as a continuing inflammatory disease of the pancreas, characterized by irreversible morphological change, and typically causing pain and permanent loss of function.

In 2016, a Mechanistic definition was incorporated which has characters of both end-stage pancreatic disease (pancreatic atrophy, fibrosis, pain syndromes, strictures, calcifications, exocrine, and endocrine insufficiency) as well as the mechanisms of disease pathogenesis in individuals with genetic, environmental, and/or other risk factors.

The central concept of the mechanistic definition involves an algorithm in a suspicious case of CP based on three features:

- **Clinical features**: Family history, characteristic pain, and features of pancreatic insufficiency.
- **Risk**: As per the TIGAR-0 risk assessment system (detailed below).
- **Biomarkers**: High amylase, lipase, triglycerides, vitamin deficiency (A, D, E, K), and exocrine function test.

Q. What are the components of the TIGAR-O checklist for the etiology of Chronic Pancreatitis?
The components of the TIGAR-O system can be enumerated as:

- T: Toxic or metabolic (Alcohol, smoking, hypertriglyceridemia, drugs)
- I: Idiopathic (Subclassified as early-onset <35 years and late-onset >35 years)

B. L. Meena · A. Roy · V. Singh (✉)
Department of Hepatology, Post Graduate Institute of Medical Education and Research, Chandigarh, Punjab, India

© The Author(s), under exclusive license to Springer Nature Singapore Pte Ltd. 2022
V. Singh, A. Roy (eds.), *Clinical Rounds in Hepatology*,
https://doi.org/10.1007/978-981-16-8448-7_23

- G: Genetic (PRSS-1, CFTR, SPINK-1)
- A: Autoimmune Pancreatitis Type 1 and 2
- R: Recurrent acute or severe pancreatitis
- O: Obstructive lesions

Q. What are the common genetic polymorphisms that are implicated in CP? In patients with Idiopathic Pancreatitis, what are the essential genetic evaluations that should be done?
Acinar cell dysfunction polymorphisms

- PRSS1 (cationic trypsinogen gene)
- CPA1 (carboxypeptidase A1 gene)
- CEL (carboxyl ester lipase) A
- SPINK1 (serine protein inhibitor Kazal type 1)
- CTRC (chymotrypsin C)

Ductal cell dysfunction polymorphisms

- CFTR (cystic fibrosis transmembrane conductance regulator)

Disease-modifying genes polymorphisms

- CASR (calcium-sensing receptor gene)
- CTRC (chymotrypsin C)
- CLDN2 locus (Claudin-2 gene locus)

Although extensive panels can be ordered in resourceful centers, however, the essential mutations that should be looked for are PRSS1, SPINK1, CFTR, and CTRC.

Q. What are the areas for scoring for assessing the severity of Chronic Pancreatitis as per the M-ANNHEIM System?
The acronym M-ANNHEIM has been used for pancreatitis with **M**ultiple risk factors-**A**lcohol consumption, **N**icotine consumption, **N**utritional factors, **H**ereditary factors, **E**fferent duct factors, **I**mmunological factors, **M**iscellaneous, and rare metabolic factors. It is used scoring system for the grading of chronic pancreatitis severity by using the following factors:

- Patient report of pain
- Pain control
- Surgical intervention
- Exocrine insufficiency
- Endocrine insufficiency

- Severe organ complications
- Morphologic status on pancreatic imaging (according to the Cambridge classification)

The severity is graded as:

- M-ANNHEIM A Minor 0–5 points
- M-ANNHEIM B Increased 6–10 points
- M-ANNHEIM C Advanced 11–15 points
- M-ANNHEIM D Marked 16–20 points
- M-ANNHEIM E Exacerbated .20 points

Q. Describe in brief the natural history of CP?

The evolution of CP is thought to be subsequent to a series of acute pancreatic injuries at the acinar level or ductal level. These events are labeled as the Sentinel Acute Pancreatitis Event (SAPE), which do not necessarily translate into clinical events. The transition into chronicity occurs in phases, although the spatial distribution is not homogenous, and there can be significant overlaps between the phases:

- Early: First 5 years characterized by recurrent episodes of pain.
- Intermediate: 5–10 years characterized by morphological changes such as pancreatic calculi, ductal strictures, and pseudocysts.
- Late stages: Usually after 10 years characterized by pancreatic exocrine insufficiency and diabetes.

Q. What is Type 3c Diabetes?

Diabetes secondary to CP is termed Type 3c diabetes, which occurs due to islet cell loss. Patients with advanced CP usually have a low body mass index compared to the classical obese type 2 diabetes phenotype. The duration of CP is the primary risk factor for the development of endocrine failure. Western literature shows that diabetes in CP occurs around 10 years after disease onset; however, Indian literature suggests an earlier onset (Talukdar R et al. Pancreatology 2013).

Q. What are the causes of pain in CP, and what are its options for management?

Causes of pain in CP include:

- Ongoing disease process
- Pancreatic pseudocyst
- Duodenal obstruction
- Biliary obstruction and cholangitis
- Development of pancreatic cancer

The options for management of pain are multiple, and the approach should be based on the WHO (World Health Organisation) Step ladder approach for pain control:

- **Analgesics**: NSAIDs, Opioids.
- **Antioxidants**: Methionine, beta carotene, selenium, vitamin C.
- **Neuromodulators**: Pregabalin.
- **Pancreatic enzyme replacement therapy**: Although frequently used in the clinical setting, a recent meta-analysis has shown a lack of efficacy with regard to analgesia with pancreatic enzyme supplementation (Yaghoobi M et al. 2016). However, PERT should be considered in patients with exocrine insufficiency to improve the complications of malnutrition.
- **Endoscopic management**: Extracorporeal shock wave lithotripsy (ESWL) with or without endoscopic retrograde cholangiopancreatography (ERCP) and stenting is currently recommended for large obstructive pancreatic ductal stones, especially those located in the head and body region. According to one study with a follow up of 2–5 years, there was complete pain relief in 68.7% of patients (Tandan et al. GIE 2013).
- **Surgical intervention**: For long-term relief of pain after first-line endoscopic approaches have been exhausted or unsuccessful.
- **TPIAT**: (Total pancreatectomy with islet auto-transplant) Should be considered only in cases of refractory pain when all other resources of pain control have been exhausted.

Q. What are the characteristics of biliary obstruction in CP?

Ans: CBD stricture may be seen in 3–46% of cases of CP (Abdullah et al., HPBS 2007) and is more commonly seen with calcific CP.

Clinical presentation:

- Incidental in 17%
- Jaundice 30–50%
- Cholangitis 10%
- Secondary biliary cirrhosis: 7.3%

Biochemical marker: ALP > 2× ULN: specific for CBD stricture
Radiological findings
Five types of bile duct stricture:

- Type I: Long retro-pancreatic stenosis (Common)
- Type II: Spincter of oddi stricture with dilated common bile duct (Common)
- Type III: Hourglass CBD stricture
- Type IV: Symptomatic of cyst/cancer
- Type V: Carcinoma of the pancreas

Q. What are the indications of biliary Drainage in Chronic Pancreatitis?

1. Symptomatic cholangitis
2. Biliary cirrhosis (Biopsy proven)
3. CBD stones along with CBD stricture
4. Progression of CBD stricture based on radiology
5. Persistent jaundice > 1 month
6. Persistent raised ALP (3XULN) > 1 month (Abdullah et al., HPBS 2007)

Q. What are the options for the management of biliary obstruction in CP?
Endoscopic intervention, either using multiple plastic stents (MPS) or a fully covered self-expanding metal stent (FCSEMS), are available modalities for managing biliary obstruction secondary to stricture in CP.

A previous study showed that a 6-month treatment with either multiple 10-Fr plastic stents or one 10-mm SEMS produces good long-term relief of biliary stricture caused by chronic pancreatitis (Haapamäki et al. Endoscopy 2014). Another recent trial has shown that endotherapy with multiple plastic stents provides similar efficacy and safety for 12-month treatment as single FCSEMS, with FCSEMS requiring fewer ERCPs over 2 years (Ramchandani et al. Gastroenterology 2021).

Further Reading

Gardner TB, et al. ACG clinical guideline: chronic pancreatitis. ACG. 2020;115(3):322–39.